For Maria, Kazimir and Dominic who generously tolerated my obsession and preoccupation and for my parents, Bob and Peg, who would have been more than a little surprised at what I have persuaded others to achieve.

Humane Prisons

Edited by

David Jones

Foreword by

Craig Haney

RADCLIFFE PUBLISHING

OXFORD • SEATTLE

Radcliffe Publishing Ltd
18 Marcham Road
Abingdon
Oxon OX14 1AA
United Kingdom
www.radcliffe-oxford.com

Electronic catalogue and worldwide online ordering facility.

British Library Cataloguing in Publication Data
A catalogue record for this book is available from the British Library.

ISBN-10 1 85775 720 3
ISBN-13 978 1 85775 720 0

Typeset by Anne Joshua & Associates, Oxford
Printed and bound by TJ International Ltd, Padstow, Cornwall

Contents

Foreword

I spend a fair amount of time inside maximum security prisons. Usually I have gone to evaluate the psychological effects of particular conditions of confinement – increasingly, in one of the 'supermax' prisons or special units that have been erected in many different parts of the United States. This process always includes interviewing a sample of prisoners who may have been adversely affected by the way they were kept or treated inside. I have been doing this for a long time – the better part of the last three decades. Whatever else can be said about this kind of activity, it has brought me into contact with a wide range of penal institutions. Talking at length with prisoners who are housed throughout the vast state and federal prison systems in the United States has also provided me with a rare opportunity to witness some of the human costs and consequences of current penal policies – to hear about the shattered lives, to see the wounded psyches and to marvel at the unexpected signs of resilience. Little that I have seen or heard has left me optimistic or hopeful about our ability to create truly 'humane prisons'. That is, not until I came upon the present, remarkable volume.

The goal of creating prisons like the ones that are described and envisioned in the chapters that follow is a daunting one. Frankly, it has become much more daunting as a result of correctional policies and perspectives that emerged over the last several decades. The United States, it could be argued, played a key role in leading the rest of the world down this pessimistic path toward a dark place in the history of corrections. It was the first modern industrial nation in recent years to strike out in an openly and exclusively punitive direction – to introduce increasingly draconian sentencing policies that greatly expanded the numbers of people who were imprisoned and the lengths of time that they stayed behind bars. It also was the first to implement a host of correspondingly harsh prison practices that abandoned any hope of accomplishing anything beyond the inevitable punishment of prison – to reject rehabilitation not only as a goal that we had failed to fully achieve but also as one not remotely worth the aspiration.

Some prison policymakers (and even some academic experts) tried to dignify this politically expedient approach to crime control by claiming that 'punishment for punishment's sake' was some kind of new correctional 'philosophy', as if the goal of locking up the most people possible for the longest time possible could be portrayed as an 'advance' in anyone's thinking. Nonetheless, despite the lack of *any* compelling evidence that spreading the pains of imprisonment could accomplish its alleged purpose – a reduction of crime that was remotely commensurate with the resources we invested in these hurtful policies – spread them we did.

It would be impossible for anyone who has not seen these changes firsthand to fully grasp or appreciate the extraordinary increase in the sheer scale of imprisonment that has occurred over the last several decades. Similarly, it would be difficult to capture in words – for people who have not felt or absorbed the depth and breadth of the transformation – how attitudes have hardened among staff members in many of these institutions, the way corrections has become a business that too often trades in human suffering, and the new matter-of-factness that characterizes the callous mistreatment occurring inside a number of penal institutions. Those of us who have lived through this period sometimes forget how significantly the atmosphere in prison and the norms of confinement have changed.

By virtue of their sheer size and the many self-justifying rationales that surround and permeate them, prisons have a way of conveying a sense of inevitability. Not only, 'this is the way things are', but 'this is they way they always have been', and, even more uncompromisingly, 'this is the way they must be, the only way they could be. . . .' Only people with long experience and good memories can give lie to these assertions, and only those with active imaginations can think past their implication.

In the face of all of this, what can the chapters that follow do to inspire hopefulness? Most of all, they contain the voices of people who *care*. They convey the insights, observations, and concerns of scholars and professionals who have refused to succumb to the 'new penology', one that my colleagues Malcolm Feeley and Jonathan Simon have described as serving a despairing and demeaning 'waste management' function. Far from succumbing, they urge us in an opposite direction. These authors are sober and realistic analysts, to be sure, yet they are also compassionate and dedicated reformers who refuse to sacrifice imagination for practicality. They seek "humane prisons" at a time in corrections history when too many others aspire only to maintain 'secure' and 'controlled' spaces – the kind of security and control that too often come at the price of humanity, it saddens me to say.

'Think Security. Get Back to Basics' were the ironic words written on large signs strategically placed throughout a large maximum security prison I toured just a short time ago in the midwestern United States. Ironic because, looking around this cruel and hostile place, it was painfully obvious that security had been its only concern. Too often, this 'basic' goal – admittedly important – dwarfs all others in the minds of many correctional policymakers, and even academic thinkers with the luxury of imagining a better future.

Not so the authors of the chapters that follow. Of course, they are realistic enough to concede that, even in humane prisons, guards and prisoners alike may still lack sufficient opportunities for meaningful activity and constructive purpose. They know that even well-treated prisoners can come out of prison seemingly fit and resilient, yet return to their 'unsettled' lifestyles – lifestyles forced on them as much by their unforgiving surroundings as any personal choices they might make about the directions they pursue. They admit that there is still a sense – pervasive in some places in spite of the humane intentions of those in charge – that the environment systematically undermines the sense of self or shared humanity among those confined inside.

Indeed, the authors are realists who lament the continued existence of prisons where fear, idleness, and callous treatment are still capable of creating or exacerbating prison madness, and ones where violence is seen by prisoners as commonplace, conventional, and even something that is expected of them. And they concede that the transfer of coping skills developed in prison – even the best of them – will rarely assist prisoners in successfully reintegrating into free society. Indeed, they know that prisoners typically re-enter a world that is not only vastly different from the one they have become accustomed to in prison, but one that, by virtue of their incarceration, has grown even more foreign and hostile to them.

Yet, despite this realism, this is a book full of honesty, of insight, of heart, and of imagination – all things that have been sorely lacking in much writing about prison policy and prison practices over the last several decades. Many of the authors are visionaries, grappling with the best ways to get from where we are to where we might – and should – be. Others are practitioners, laboring to make sense of whether and when their good intentions can be translated into actual policies and practices that reflect their humane values. Part of the inspiration that readers will glean from this book comes directly from the boldness and authenticity of the quest – to create 'humane prisons' at a time when so many others have given up on the goal! The seriousness with which each author engages this challenge is unmistakable.

In addition to the sheer inspiration, many of the ideas that follow have direct, practical applications that can be pursued in other less enlightened prison systems. For example, American readers will find the prison inspection process used in British prison to be remarkable and worthy of emulation, not only because of the 'robust independence' with which it proceeds, but also the sophisticated perspective that it brings to bear. Indeed, British prisons are inspected regularly and without warning, and the results – on the culture and decency of the institution – are a matter of public record. In addition, prison inspectors do confidential, random surveys of all prisoners before each inspection, and have a comparative base – both between different prisons and for the same prisons over time – that allows for a measure of performance from the prisoners' point of view. The inspectors' goal, explicitly stated, is to determine whether prisoners are being housed safely, treated with respect, engaged in purposeful activity, and being prepared for their return to the community. There is certainly much more to this story, and I should not belabor it here, but the value of such a straightforward intelligent practice seems difficult to dispute.

The therapeutic community perspective that is reflected in many of the chapters is one important approach to creating humane prisons. Of course, it is not the only one. Legitimate concerns have been expressed about the logic and practice of therapeutic prisons, and they are acknowledged here. Crime is not necessarily caused by the damaged psyches of its perpetrators, and psychotherapeutic interventions in prison do not necessarily prepare prisoners for the transition to the free world or assist them in overcoming the socioeconomic and other barriers they will confront there. Moreover, even a good idea – or otherwise effective intervention – can be badly or poorly implemented in the difficult environment of prison. And, as one of the authors wisely reminds us, the inherent tendency for treatment (or any intervention) to become punitive when it is 'married to structures of control' must not be overlooked.

Yet, there is still something to be said for an analysis of these total institutions that recognizes the ways in which the extreme and sometimes extremely cruel, punitive treatment to which prisoners are exposed interferes with and impedes personal growth of any kind, therapeutic or otherwise. And there is certainly something to be gained from listening to authors who understand that the best way to create a sustainable social order (inside prison and beyond) is to address people's basic needs, and hearing the voices of people who unfailingly respect the moral obligation to treat prisoners humanely.

Wisdom, intelligent and compassionate analysis, and imagination have all been lacking in much of the discourse and debate over the future of imprisonment in the modern world. Thankfully, they are in abundance in the pages that follow. Perhaps this contribution will begin the long overdue re-opening of a badly needed dialogue and discussion. It could not have come at a better time.

Craig Haney
Professor of Psychology
University of California
August 2006

About the editor

David Jones is a Consultant Adult Psychotherapist in Forensic Psychiatry, East London and City NHS Trust and has worked with police staff and with traumatised refugees. He formerly led the Assessment Unit at the therapeutic prison, HMP Grendon. His first edited volume was *Working With Dangerous People: the psychotherapy of violence*, also published by Radcliffe.

About the contributors

Peter Bennett gained a PhD at the School of Oriental and African Studies, University of London, in 1983. He has served as a governor grade in the Prison Service of England and Wales for some 23 years, including as governing governor of Nottingham, Wellingborough and Grendon/Springhill. He has published a book and numerous articles on social anthropological and penal themes.

Ernest L Cowles PhD is currently the Director of the Institute for Social Research and Professor of Sociology at the California State University, Sacramento. Prior to accepting his present position, he directed a similar research institute at the University of Illinois for ten years. In addition to his background as an academic and researcher, Dr Cowles served as a probation and parole officer and prison psychologist early in his career, and later returned to the 'real world' of prison to serve as a deputy director of a state department of corrections. In addition to an ongoing abiding interest in correctional issues, his recent research has involved substance abuse, drug enforcement, information systems, and human services delivery in healthcare. Dr Cowles' writings appear in a number of books, journal articles, research monographs and reports. He holds a PhD in Criminology from the Florida State University.

Kimmett Edgar is Head of Research at the Prison Reform Trust. He was formerly Senior Research Officer at the Oxford Centre for Criminological Research.

Erwin James was born to Scottish parents in Clevedon in Somerset in 1957. A family lifestyle described as 'brutal and rootless' by a prison psychologist following the death of his mother when James was seven, led to a limited formal education. He gained his first criminal conviction aged 10 and was taken into care in Yorkshire aged 11. His teenage and early adult years were spent drifting, living with extended family members, and often sleeping rough. He worked in various labouring jobs, but also committed relatively petty, mostly acquisitive but occasionally violent, crimes, (criminal damage, common assault). His directionless way of life continued, including several years in the French Foreign Legion, until 1984, when he was jailed for life. In prison he took a degree course with the Open University majoring in History and graduated in 1994. His first article for a national newspaper, the *Independent*, appeared in 1994. He won first prize in the annual Koestler Awards for prose in 1995. He also wrote for prison magazines. His first article in the *Guardian* appeared in 1998. He began writing a regular column, entitled *A Life Inside*, in the *Guardian* in 2000. A collection of his columns *A Life Inside, a prisoner's notebook*, was published in 2003. A follow-up, *The Home Stretch, from prison to parole*, was published in April 2005. Both were published by Atlantic Books. James was released from prison in August 2004, and continues to write for the *Guardian*. He also works as a development manager for a national charity. Erwin James lives on the coast.

Tilman Kluttig is a clinical psychologist and psychotherapist. In clinical practice since 1986, he has been since 1997 senior clinical psychologist in the Department for Forensic Psychiatry and Psychotherapy of the Reichenau Mental Hospital and head of a ward for forensic psychotherapy. He trained as a psychodrama therapist, family therapist, cognitive-behavioural therapist and in psychoanalytical psychotherapy for patients with psychotic disorders. Since 2002 he has been a member of the executive board of the International Association for Forensic Psychotherapy.

Terry A Kupers, MD, MSP, practices psychiatry in Oakland, California, and is Institute Professor at The Wright Institute. He has worked or consulted in community mental health agencies since completing his psychiatric training at UCLA and The Tavistock Institute. He has testified in over 20 class action lawsuits about jail and prison conditions, the adequacy of correctional mental health services, the toxic effects of isolated confinement (supermax) and rape of prisoners. He has served as consultant to Human Rights Watch, Amnesty International and Stop Prisoner Rape. His four books include *Public Therapy: The Practice of Psychotherapy in the Public Mental Health Clinic* (1981, Free Press) and *Prison Madness: The Mental Health Crisis Behind Bars and What We Must Do About It* (Jossey-Bass/Wiley, 1999). He is also co-editor of *Prison Masculinities* (Temple University Press, 2001). He is Contributing Editor of *Correctional Mental Health Report*; and he received a 2005 Exemplary Psychiatrist Award from the National Alliance for the Mentally Ill.

Liz McLure is a qualified Group Analyst with a background in Nursing and Education. She works as a psychotherapist both at HMP Grendon and in private practice.

Sunny Marriner is the founder and coordinator of the Young Women At Risk (YWAR) Program at the Sexual Assault Support Centre of Ottawa. YWAR provides counselling, support, and advocacy for marginalised, criminalised and incarcerated survivors of sexual assault and abuse from a human rights, women's equality, anti-oppression framework. Her areas of concentration include criminal justice, sexual exploitation and youth imprisonment. She is a regular guest lecturer on issues of access to justice, punishment and the criminalisation of victims of abuse. Her publications include work on the use of psychiatric drugs with young women, and analyses of media reporting of sexual assault.

Dawn Moore is an Assistant Professor in the Law Department at Carleton University. She has written on contemporary penal issues in Canada including prison privatisation, therapy in prisons and the 'punitive turn' in Canadian punishment. She is currently working on a book project that explores the rise and current practices of penal addiction treatment in Canada with a particular focus on drug treatment courts.

Mark Morris is a doctor, psychiatrist and psychoanalyst. He trained at the Cassel Hospital in London, worked as Director of Therapy in Grendon Prison, at the Portman Clinic and with the High Secure Prison Directorate. He now leads the medium secure Kneesworth House Personality Disorder Service.

Anne Owers has been Her Majesty's Chief Inspector of Prisons in England and Wales since August 2001. She was previously (from 1992) Director of JUSTICE, an all-party human rights and law reform organisation and the British section of the International Commission of Jurists. From 1981–92, she worked at the Joint Council for the Welfare of Immigrants (a national organisation undertaking casework and policy work on immigration and asylum), first as research and policy officer, then as General Secretary (from 1986). Before that, she undertook a variety of research and community work in Africa and South London, focusing on race relations and legal advice work. She has written various articles and publications on human rights, prisons and asylum.

Kathy Page is a novelist and short story writer, born in the UK but currently living on the west coast of Canada with her husband and two children. Her fifth novel, *The Story of My Face*, was longlisted for the Orange Prize in 2002. She has worked as a Writer in Residence in a variety of universities and in other settings, including a Norfolk fishing village, and, in 1992, HMP Nottingham, a Category B men's prison; her latest novel *Alphabet*, 2004, arose out of that experience. Her website can be visited at www.Kathy Page.info.

Lorna A Rhodes teaches medical anthropology, the anthropology of institutions and ethnographic research methods at the University of Washington. She is the author of *Emptying Beds: The Work of an Emergency Psychiatric Unit* (University of California Press, 1991) and *Total Confinement: Madness and Reason in the Maximum Security Prison* (University of California Press, 2004). She has also published a number of articles about supermax prisons, including most recently 'Changing the Subject: Conversation in Supermax' in *Cultural Anthropology* (2005). Rhodes was medical anthropology editor of *Social Science and Medicine* from 1989 to 1993 and currently serves on several editorial boards, including *Medical Anthropology* and the *Howard Journal of Criminal Justice*.

Hans Toch is Distinguished Professor at the School of Criminal Justice, University at Albany, State University of New York in the USA. He holds a PhD in psychology from Princeton University. He has published extensively. His last books are *Acting Out* (with Ken Adams) and *Stress in Policing*. Among his other books are *Living in Prison*, *Violent Men*, and *Mosaic of Despair: Human Breakdowns in Prison*.

Sarah Tucker is a Wing Therapist at HMP Grendon. She is Group Analyst and Honorary Research Fellow at the Royal College of Psychiatrist's Research and Training Unit. She is a member of the Association of Therapeutic Communities Steering Group and on the editorial collective of *Therapeutic Communities: The International Journal for Therapeutic and Supportive Organisations*.

Fiona Warren is Lecturer in Psychology at the University of Surrey. Her research interests are in personality disorders, self-harm and therapeutic communities. She worked for some years on studies of the effectiveness of Henderson Hospital NHS residential therapeutic community, and recently conducted a review of treatments for personality disorders for the Home Office and an analysis of therapeutic community research in prisons for HM Prison Service.

Adrian Worrall has led the development of five quality networks at the Royal College of Psychiatrists Research Unit: the Clinical Governance Support Service (CGSS); the Quality Network for In-patient Child and Adolescent Mental health Services (QNIC); Children and Adolescents Mental Health Services (CAMHS); the Quality Improvement Network for Multi-agency (QINMAC); Community of Communities (CC); and the ECT Accreditation Service (ECTAS). These use a clinical audit model within a peer-support network. Each year standards are agreed then applied in self- and external peer-review.

He has developed eight sets of standards, in consultation with staff and service users, for different levels and speciality areas of mental health services, including standards for the Department of Health to support the commissioning of services. He previously managed the National In-patient Child and Adolescent Psychiatry Study (NICAPS) and worked on a report for ministers commissioned via the Clinical Standards Advisory Group (CSAG) on services for people with depression. He is interested in programme evaluation and is now leading the evaluation of a major Modernisation Agency initiative. He has co-edited a Gaskell book on clinical governance in mental health and learning disability services and is now editing a book on European therapeutic communities.

The quality of mercy is not strain'd,
It droppeth as the gentle rain from heaven
Upon the place beneath: it is twice blest;
It blesseth him that gives and him that takes:
'Tis mightiest in the mightiest: it becomes
The throned monarch better than his crown;
His sceptre shows the force of temporal power,
The attribute to awe and majesty,
Wherein doth sit the dread and fear of kings;
But mercy is above this sceptred sway;
It is enthroned in the hearts of kings,
It is an attribute to God himself;
And earthly power doth then show likest God's
When mercy seasons justice.

The Merchant of Venice
William Shakespeare
Act IV: Scene 1

'The first time I voted for the death penalty, I thought of the law as majestic and that there was very little chance of a mistake. Then you grow up. Look at the DNA evidence – you realize that people can make terrible mistakes. . . . Times change. I never thought I'd vote against the death penalty. But I've come to realize that no one's perfect, including judges and juries.'

New York Assemblyman Joseph R Lentol
Washington Post 13 April 2005
www.washingtonpost.com/wp-dyn/articles/A47871-2005Apr12.html

Acknowledgements

A book made in this way demands trust and patience from authors. Many of them have never met me and I am most grateful for the way that we have been able to negotiate over the course of a year. Colleagues at HMP Grendon have always been tolerant of my preoccupations and forgiving when I have over-stepped the mark. I owe a particular debt to Nigel Hopton who has diligently kept me updated about the increasing level of bureaucratic intrusion and the reducing level of privilege that prisoners experience. Martin Groves instructed me in the skill required to invigorate and train a group of prison officers. We would have had a great chapter had time allowed and tape recorders worked properly! Finally my editor, Maggie Pettifer, has continued to support and encourage me while keeping me on track with great delicacy.

Introduction

Why humane prisons?

I remember lying in bed one morning in 1991 listening to the radio. The first Iraq war was coming to an end and the Iraqi army was trailing out of Kuwait on the way home. This particular soundtrack was a recording of young American men in an orgy of excitement at the explosions they were producing below. Like a scene in a computer game they were able to cause the moving trucks in their sights to burst into flame and disappear. However, the ecstasy was produced by the awareness that real human beings were being snuffed out. This chilling experience reminded me of what people are capable of if they are able to distance themselves sufficiently from the humanity of the other and simultaneously invest this same other with qualities of evil. This is the problem we face in the field of criminal justice. As our feelings become polarised about criminals so it is possible to lose sight of humane values and, more pragmatically, of the benefit that can accrue to individual and community through reducing the criminalising effects of imprisonment and redirecting the antisocial and self-destructive tendencies of many prisoners.

Our book began in optimistic frame of mind. While it would be accurate to report that the optimism reduced somewhat during the period of its preparation, the sense of urgency that I felt at the beginning remains. The intention was always to provide clear examples of good practice as well as drawing attention to the real difficulties faced in this field of work. I think that we have succeeded in doing this by drawing upon a wide range of experience from Europe and North America. I am truly proud of the way this book has been created by people of tremendous experience from across North America and Europe.

Background

In the year just passed, the thousandth execution since the death penalty was reintroduced in 1976 has been performed in the United States. By the time this book is published I would expect that another 40 or more convicts will have been legally killed through a variety of methods. The largest proportion of these executions, more than one-third, will have occurred in one state, Texas, while the largest state, California, has executed eleven.

Meanwhile the number of men incarcerated continues to increase, with highest numbers seen in the United States of America, followed by the Russian Federation. The rate of incarceration in the USA is seven times that of Germany (ICPS, 2005) or ten times if Texas is used as the comparison state. The rate of increase in the United States and in England is similar. These figures and the startling variation across national and state borders are indicative of the influence of social, cultural and political forces upon rates of both incarceration and execution. The reasons for these developments are complex and subject to much debate. (Garland; Zimring; Monkkonen; Whitman; all 2005). Most striking is the difference between mainland Europe and the USA and to a slighter extent the UK, and this difference is characterised by a drift towards increasing harshness of punishment and level of degradation of offenders in America.

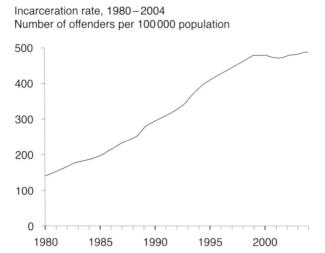

Incarceration rate, 1980–2004
Number of offenders per 100 000 population

Figure A Incarceration rate, 1980–2004
Source: US Department of Justice 2005: www.ojp.usdoj.gov/bjs/correct.htm

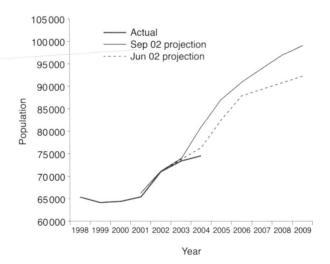

Figure B Prison population projections 2005–2011 01/05 England and Wales
Source: de Silva (2005)

Humane prisons

This book acknowledges these social and political trends, particularly the part played by social deprivation and racism, and the importance of continuing to understand them. But the book is not simply an academic discourse; instead it attempts to provide ideas, examples and models for others to use, add to or challenge. It does not fall easily into parts but flows following the introductory chapter by **Hans Toch**. There is no division between theory and practice: rather all of the authors have been or still are deeply involved in work related to the field. Professor Toch, with the benefit of his accumulated wisdom, warns of the danger of high expectations and of the importance of being honest in the presentation of our work and the results arising from it. The next two chapters, by **Kathy Page** and **Erwin James**, provide uniquely personal accounts of their time spent in the English prison system. Although they come from quite different backgrounds the similarity of their accounts is quite uncanny. Page, a novelist, was employed as a Writer in Residence for a year. The freshness of her eye conveys brilliantly the mixture of drabness, boredom, energy and excitement that is to be found in prisons. From the opposite direction, James, who spent over twenty years as a prisoner, illustrates the remarkable resilience of the human spirit. His first-hand account presents a picture of a dangerous environment where the first priority was to ensure your safety. For some, like James, the tortuous and lengthy negotiations through the lifer system can bring some opportunities for self-development. For others, those more vulnerable, the risk is of bullying, a slide into drug addiction and mental illness.

The next three chapters consider mental states and their relationship with imprisonment. **David Jones** argues that the total complex around prison systems, from political structures to prison wing, is intrinsically unstable and moves between different degrees of psychopathology. He looks at the way in which systems and individuals may be caught up in these states and suggests that Correctional Departments should take positive steps to moderate the effects of such unconscious dynamics. **Terry Kupers** describes in stark and alarming detail how many prison practices can have a direct and serious effect on the mental health of convicts. Having described the 'recipe' for creating madness in prisons he is in a position to reverse the process. The question of violence in prisons is addressed by **Kimmet Edgar**. Based upon eight years of research, this chapter explores the concept of social order, discusses the sources and effects of conflict and proposes a conflict centred strategy for reducing violence.

The next two chapters by **Lorna Rhodes** and **Mark Morris** are both concerned with conditions of very high security, The Supermaximum (Supermax) in the United States and the Close Supervision Centres in the United Kingdom. Both chapters are based upon extensive personal experience and research describing places of confinement that are extraordinarily restricting and demoralising. The two sites clearly differ, making the comparisons rich and stimulating.

Ernest Cowles is an expert in matters relating to gangs in prison and treatment conditions. His chapter highlights the difficulties that usually exist in running successful treatment programmes in prisons and the confusion that can sometimes develop around the difference between punishment and treatment. He argues for systemic change within prisons so that effective treatments can flourish.

The position of prisons for women has been under-reported and, arguably, under-discussed. **Sunny Marriner** and **Dawn Moore** challenge the complacency of the 'too few to count' rhetoric and argue that women live in the shadows of the prison system. They are concerned about the bias contained in risk assessment schemes and the moral judgments contained in treatment programmes. These structures that appear designed to promote more liberal settings often disguise a more regressive approach. They argue powerfully that the case has been made for sweeping change many times over the past two decades and that recommendations have either been ignored or only partially implemented.

Running a prison is no easy matter. Prisons are large organisations with a large budget and employing many staff. The Governor is the fulcrum who determines the direction that a prison takes, within certain limits. The pressure comes from many directions, as **Peter Bennett** describes so richly in his chapter. Bennett has had the good fortune to manage a variety of interesting prisons during his career and is now in charge of a prison with a particularly good reputation. His chapter is a fascinating perspective from an anthropologist situated within his project.

Staff are the most valuable resource in prisons and frequently they are ill supported and underpaid. Staff work and survive better if they receive regular support and supervision. **Liz McLure** and **Tilman Kluttig**, from a German perspective, write about the support and supervision that is given to uniformed prison staff (guards or wardens) as well as to other professionally trained staff who work therapeutically with highly challenging serious offenders. Most of these offenders would be considered untreatable, even unmanageable, in other settings. In this setting, where men are treated with respect and afforded a greater degree of control than is usual, infractions of prison rules, such as violence and drug use, are greatly reduced and rates of recidivism are also less than would be expected. There is a cost to this, of course. While the work is more enjoyable and rewarding for staff, they are compelled to listen to highly disturbing material and to experience the complex and often perverse psychodynamics of men who will most probably have experienced a history of terrible physical or sexual abuse before going on to commit their own horrific crimes.

The final three chapters take a quite different approach. **Fiona Warren** tackles the highly problematic matter of cost. Politicians do not like spending money on criminals. They believe, probably correctly, that there are no votes in spending money on prisoners. However, this is almost certainly a false economy, since making substantial advances in reducing reoffending rates would bring massive overall savings. It is a difficult matter to prove and is an area ripe for research. Warren uses her experience of the successful cost benefit analysis of the Henderson Hospital to argue the case for Humane Prisons. Finally, **Sarah Tucker** and **Adrian Worrall** and **Anne Owers** present descriptions of different ways of bringing about and maintaining change within organisations. Tucker and Worrall developed a highly innovative structure of peer review, originally for therapeutic communities, across a range of different fields. This then merged with a prison service accreditation system to provide a regular, sensitive and systematic approach to measuring the quality of the therapeutic community. The Chief Inspector of Prisons has a far wider brief and in many ways a much more difficult job. The task is to visit every prison, on a planned and unplanned basis, regularly and to provide a comprehensive report. Anne Owers' chapter provides a revealing insight into the detailed workings of a prison system.

References

de Silva N (2005) *Prison Population Projections 2005–2011*. HMSO, London. Available at: www.homeoffice.gov.uk/rds/pdfs05/hosb0105.pdf.

Garland D (2005) Capital punishment and American culture. *Punishment and Society*. 7(4): 347–76.

International Centre for Prison Studies (ICPS) (2005) www.kcl.ac.uk/depsta/rel/icps/worldbrief/highest_to_lowest_rates.php.

Monkkonen E (2005) Reaction to David Garland on capital punishment. *Punishment and Society*. 7(4) 385–7.

Whitman JQ (2005) Response to Garland. *Punishment and Society*. 7(4) 389–96.

Zimring FE (2005) Path dependence, culture and state-level execution policy. *Punishment and Society*. 7(4) 377–84.

Chapter 1

Is there a future for humane imprisonment?

Hans Toch

To an observer from Mars, our prisons may look silly and ineffective. This fact need not surprise us because our prisons reflect our state of ignorance and our sense of impotence. We feel constrained to run the sorts of prisons we do because of our failure to understand most maladaptive and violent behaviour, and our inability to deal with it. Given our unconscious awareness of our deficits, we have largely fallen back on strategies of containment and control.

To be sure, there have been some occasions along the way in which we have improved our knowledge of violent offenders and our skill in dealing with them, and have been able to devise and operate different types of institutions. It would be nice to presume that such ventures would be bound to prosper and multiply, but this has often not been the case. Sadly, history is redolent with brave but ultimately unsuccessful experiments with enlightened and decent penological practices – many of these being ahead of their time and of ours. I think that it behoves us to consider these debacles with a dispirited yet open mind, so that we can hopefully learn from them.

The key question is: Why were so many admirable experiments so consistently short-lived? Some observers, of course, believe that this question is silly, because they define 'humane imprisonment' as an oxymoronic juxtaposition of incompatible objectives. Other observers prefer to see most past (and future) prison innovations as naive expressions of ivy-towered idealism, or as the unreplicable and predictably evanescent handiwork of one-off charismatic leaders. This latter charge may especially ring true because the chronologies frequently involve coinciding life cycles of interventions and their founders.

A very different type of contention has been that humane imprisonment by its nature offends public sensibilities, violating expectations and challenging cherished assumptions. Given this contingency, it becomes a mere matter of time for the resistances that the experiments invite to gel into an organised opposition. This chain of events tends to particularly appeal to sadder-but-wiser partisans of humane confinement, because it serves to explain their own failures, and those of their friends. It also happens to be another plausible narrative, in that many correctional interventions have unquestionably fallen victim to political forces carefully plotting their demise.

Aiming for the Achilles Heel

The environment of humane imprisonment can be compared to a besieging army, whose chances of prevailing are facilitated by vulnerabilities in its target. Those who operate humane prison programmes are consequently well advised to engage in continuous self-review and unsparing self-critiques. It is important to keep in mind that innocuous inconsistencies in programme design or imperfections in implementation are far from uncommon in pioneering interventions, as are occasional errors in judgment. But we need to recognise that such human failings and foibles become exploitable if they are ignored or swept under the rug. Assaults on pioneering enterprises have tended to highlight their shortcomings and make them salient, but these outcomes have been facilitated where programmes were awkwardly or stubbornly defended. Immodestly touted programmes can be made to look silly where attention is drawn to ways in which they fall short of their advertised perfection.

It is of course inviting for anyone who is ridiculed or skewered to blame his or her misfortune on others, such as whistleblowers who relay misinformation to ill-intentioned confederates. But publicised shortcomings have often come to light through the advent of critical incidents of the sort that are bound to occur when one is dealing with high-risk clients. Moreover, information leaks point to unresolved dissension or live disharmony in one's ranks. An intervention that is truly innovative or distinctive cannot afford to be a house divided. If a programme does stand out it can expect scrutiny, and it must strive to earn the loyalty and dedication of its staff in order to weather its predictably turbulent environment. This means that the way such a programme is organised and the way it is run can be as important as its content. Most humane settings in corrections happen to be organised democratically, which gives them a head start in this regard: organisational theory tells us that one can best engender loyalty in an organisation through participative management and shared decision-making, so that staff (and inmates, in the case of prison programmes) can develop a sense of ownership and a feeling of having a stake in the welfare and survival of the community they have helped to shape.

Promoting inclusiveness

Because pioneering programmes require solidarity in their ranks, they need to avoid anything that resembles a class or caste system. The staff of such programmes must therefore never be organised in a way that treats some as second-class citizens or makes others feel that they are relegated to the fringes of the operation. This caution sounds painfully elementary, but can be lost sight of when decisions are made about what to do with uniformed personnel, and about the role that one wants them to play. It is amazing how often it is forgotten that prison officers as a group tend to invite being unfairly stereotyped. And though many of the officers we might have encountered in mainstream prisons may have appeared hard-nosed or custody-oriented, we must realise that this would not be so because they were born with a security-prone chromosome or custodial gene. We must keep in mind that if our prisons did not have prison officers, we would be forced to invent them. Uniformed staff happen to be the front-line of prisons on a 24/7 basis. While dedicated humanists like ourselves have ambled in and out of institutions on convenient weekday shifts, it is prison officers who have been faithfully manning the fort and have acted as our most reliable and multifarious resource.

As front-line staff, officers are by nature generalists, who acquire their job-orientation and skills through training and on-the-job involvement. Where we engender appropriate training and on-the-job involvements there is no reason why in humane (as opposed to traditional or inhumane) prisons, corrections officers cannot play a prized and prominent role. In fact, in treatment-oriented or community-oriented programmes, the officers' role can be particularly enhanced and enriched. And while job enrichment is desirable both from the officers' perspective and ours, there is no uniform direction it need take, so there is considerable room for humanistic variety. The enriched or enhanced attributes of the humane officers' role are thus likely to vary from one progressive setting to another. However, some common denominators are also needed to survive. Prison officers could thus become more specialised in special programmes without relinquishing their 'basic' custodial functions and responsibilities.

The reliance on officers as front-line staff may also help us to build bridges to the remainder of the system. No matter how much top-down sponsorship a progressive programme may enjoy, it must still earn acceptance to legitimise its operation. In the process of defining itself and projecting its own identity, it must therefore try to acknowledge and accommodate goals of those elsewhere in the organisation. A new, innovative programme must take care not to overstate the significance of its uniqueness. If an intervention can do what other settings are not doing, it has a right to draw attention to this fact, and to hope that it will be valued by virtue of being both different and compatible, and of being able to contribute to the rest of the system because it can do what others cannot do or would rather not be doing.

Being a law unto oneself

The most frequent threats to the survival of humane settings do not derive from attacks on their core goals, but have to do with ancillary or tangential concerns, related to the way rules are made and privileges and penalties are dispensed. Innovative programmes have most often been disrupted or discontinued because of the allegation that they afforded their clients an unseemly privileged existence or exempted them from universally applicable rules. We can anticipate risk wherever a programme emphasises the discretionary nature of its decision-making, which in one fell swoop can irritate both prison administrators and critics from the left and the right. In the course of such jurisdictional controversies, the contribution a programme makes – which may be invaluable and substantial – can be overlooked or unattended to. Questions of boundaries between systems and subsystems frequently end up being couched in blunt and non-negotiable terms. It may of course be a truism that in the pursuit of organisational congruence it takes two to tango, but a prison entity must keep in mind that one cannot try to lead in a dance where one's partner is an 800-pound gorilla. Sadder-and-wiser prison reformer Peter Scharf (the co-originator of an ill-fated inmate community), ruefully made this point when he observed that:

[Inmates] can only *request privileges*; they cannot demand the *right* to democratic participation. As long as the inmates accede to the administration's wishes, everything runs smoothly. When there is a difference of opinion . . .the prison administration usually wins.

(Scharf, 1980, pp. 97–8).

With respect to therapeutic communities in prison, Scharf emphasised that:

The democracy of the prison therapeutic community is always a democracy within a larger correctional bureaucracy, ultimately subject to its laws, rules, jurisdictions and norms. In this context, the democracy of a prison therapeutic community is in a tenuous position, subject to powerful forces beyond its control. Such forces must be faced, because democratic participation represents a central element in the prison therapeutic community, both as an ideal in itself, and as a means toward social cohesion and group solidarity (p. 98).

Elliott Barker, who was a redoubtable pioneer in the therapeutic-community movement, made a similar cautionary observation, and listed the following version of this doctrine as one of his guiding principles:

The other side of the issue of receiving support up the line is to give support up the line. It is essential that the authority to whom the program innovator reports be kept totally informed of all matters that may potentially create difficulties. It is clear that the program innovator must earn the confidence of those by whom he is employed. This requires a working partnership in which the principal innovator is competent and conscientious with regard to the difficulties one can get an employer into, and the employer, on the other hand, is sufficiently mature to take reasonable risks, confident that the long-term benefits outweigh the inevitable short-term problems.

(Barker, 1980, p. 77)

The same caution was retrospectively voiced by Studt, Messinger and Wilson, in a book-length obituary entitled *C-Unit: Search for Community in Prison* (1968). In this book, the authors pointed out that 'any successful resocialising community must give high priority to designing its relationship with the higher authorities who determine its fate' (p. 278). C-Unit ultimately failed to achieve a mutually satisfactory relationship of this kind. In alluding to this failure, the authors laid the blame on correctional administrators, complaining that 'the [C-unit] community was never permitted to design its institutions for control in congruence with the values espoused in its welfare institutions' (p. 280). And with respect to the question of whose obligation it may have been to adjust or conform to whom, Studt, Messinger and Wilson (1968) unrepentedly declared that:

Evaluation . . . leads directly to questions about the ability of the larger systems in C-Unit's environment to support the process they had authorized. It seems clear in retrospect that the major flaw in the original plan was to leave unspecified the implicit commitments of [the prison] and the Department of Corrections when they established a small subsystem charged with initiating organisational change . . . Throughout the life of the C-Unit program, upper administration appeared to assume that the Project, once authorized, could maintain the change process within the confines of its relatively tiny inmate–staff community without calling on its organisational environment for reciprocal changes. [The prison] and the

Department of Corrections . . .were apparently totally unprepared for the fact that changing the role of the inmate in the C-Unit community would call for corresponding changes in the role performance of all employees in the system, including both the institution and the Department of Corrections, that directly affected the development of the C-Unit program (p. 285).

The devil may lie in problematic details

C-Unit ended up springing some demands on its environment that proved unacceptable to its sponsors, but even experiments that are carefully designed can overlook procedural details that in retrospect augur controversy. The following specification of goals, for example, which was promulgated in 1927, happens to hold a hint of what eventually became a problem. The preambular Statement (for the Norfolk Colony in Massachusetts) was a model of its kind, overwhelmingly enlightened and prescient, but in passing alluded to a modified approach to disciplinary sanctions – one that some eventually charged augured an invitation to anarchy, and others saw as an opening to abuses of power. The passage read:

> Each man is looked upon as an individual with individual needs and problems and with latent possibilities for good to be given such consideration as will tend toward his ultimate recovery.
>
> To this end administrative organisation and living conditions within the institution are made to approximate as nearly as may be in a prison the atmosphere and spirit of a normal community . . . and the forces of restraint and punishment, *excepts as these may be used as a method of treatment* or institutional discipline, are subordinate.
>
> (Commons, 1940, p. 3)

The originator of the Norfolk Prison Colony, Howard Gill, was surprised when he encountered resistance from his subordinates in implementing his conception of therapeutic sanctions. The ambivalence of staff members, however, reached the point where in practice disciplinary enforcement in the prison often became unpredictably inconsistent. According to the official history of the Norfolk Colony:

> It is customary in older prisons to rule that similar infractions will always have the same punishments. It is a justice that the men understand and prison authorities believe in. Mr. Gill waded into this placid water saying that uniformity was not synonymous with equality or justice. Punishment should be meted out to suit the criminal and not the crime, an attitude which the majority of the staff at Norfolk, even after six years, did not swallow. Thus we find that the old conceptions were upset and yet the new conceptions were only partially adopted.
>
> (Yahkub, 1940, p. 97)

The historian David Rothman confirmed that Gill's advocacy of individualised indeterminate punitive dispositions was troubling to many of his staff. He quoted a statement from Norfolk's chief psychologist, for example, who contended that:

> Our task is to avoid antagonism by having a few definitive rules, the infractions of which are immediately and automatically met with by punishments which tend to be definite . . . It is only by a system of definite and automatic punishments that the men can be convinced that there is justice at Norfolk and in the world.
>
> (cit. Rothman, 2002, p. 409)

Rothman maintained that in the course of achieving compromise, a system may have evolved which embodied the worst of two opposing positions:

> The principle of indeterminacy was sacrificed, and a floor was set for punishment, but no ceiling. All sentences to the jail at Norfolk were for no less than thirty days, with release allowed only after a change of heart was certified by the disciplinary committee, and the superintendent himself. In defence of this procedure Gill announced that those in the lock-up 'are to be considered as special problem cases for the casework department. It is the responsibility of the casework department to see that no opportunity for rehabilitation is overlooked for this group' (ibid.).

As one might predict, the inmate-beneficiaries of Howard Gill's so-called 'opportunities for rehabilitation' proved unappreciative (to say the least), and became increasingly resentful as prevailing terms of confinement tended to escalate. In the words of the staff member who worked directly with one of the groups of confinees: 'These men had developed an attitude of such bitterness and antagonism toward the institution as a result of this segregation in a group of "outcasts" that rediagnosis and casework seemed impossible (pp. 411–12).' Another staff member opined during the same period: 'The question is, shall Norfolk become a "penal opportunity school" (with emphasis at least as much on the "penal" as on the "opportunity"), or shall it develop into a treatment institution?' (Rothman, 2002, p. 413).

The demise of the Norfolk experiment was due to a combination of factors, including the unloading on the institution of problematic prisoners that it was not set up to handle, meaning that: 'Gill was forced to accept large numbers of inmates who became disciplinary problems but could not be transferred out' (Serrill, 1982, p. 31). The Norfolk Colony at that point was clearly not equipped with behaviour-management strategies that would permit it to deal effectively with individuals who persistently violated the rules. This defect proved fateful, but was no reflection on Gill's overall design, which conceivably may have been 'the best hope of a whole generation of prison reformers' (Serrill, 1982, p.25). In point of fact, 'whatever the ultimate value of Gill's ideas about casework and rehabilitation of inmates, it can be said with certainty that he never really got a chance to test them' (Serrill, 1982, p. 30).

What happens after the honeymoon ends?

Many progressive experiments have been snuffed out in the prime of their organisational lives, but the termination of one's programme can also resemble an act of euthanasia, ratifying a process that has been taking place over time. If we carefully review the career of defunct correctional interventions we can sometimes locate early and incipient indications of decline, with an ensuing process of more or less gradual erosion.

Almost every intervention opens with a brief honeymoon period, in which it is apt to appear happy and successful. During this time, observers will record that the level of dedication, motivation, and commitment of staff members in the programme is impressively high, as is the involvement and enthusiasm of its inmates. Such ebullience is predictably hard to sustain over long periods, but the challenge for those who institute any new venture is to retain as much of its initial momentum as long as they can, because running an enterprise that has integrity requires sustained effort and hard work by everyone concerned.

A recent prison experiment that has stood out for what its many admirers described as an over-extended honeymoon was the Barlinnie Special Unit (BSU) of the Scottish Prison Service, which opened its doors in February 1973, and received consistently panegyrical coverage until the date of its dissolution in 1995. During the first years of its life, the Barlinnie Special Unit was unquestionably 'one of the most imaginative and enlightened experiments in penal history' (Kennedy, 1982, p. 5). The BSU had been created as a therapeutic community, to be staffed by social therapists, working with the most notorious and violent prisoners in the Scottish system, who had mostly been languishing in solitary segregation. The BSU succeeded in addressing the longstanding patterns of acting-out behaviour of these prisoners, but also unleashed amazing untapped potential in some of its charges, graduating a sculptor and writer, and nourishing inmate-poets and playwrights.

Over time, the word 'therapeutic' in characterisations of the BSU came to lose its salience, while the word 'community' retained its ascendance. This re-emphasis reflected a reorientation in the Unit's staffing and regime, the core of which, however, continued to consist of regularly scheduled community meetings and specially scheduled meetings and group sessions of prisoners and staff. These assemblages had been designed to promote the in-depth exploration of daily problems of communal living and to foster interpersonal skills and maturation among the inmates. These experiences were consonant with the original mission of the BSU, and it was assumed that the prescribed activities were religiously taking place. Such was, in fact, the impression that was being conveyed by admiring acolytes writing about the BSU over the years.

In reality, however, there had been considerable slippage, and staff–inmate encounters in the Unit had become infrequent and perfunctory. Eventually, it had become inescapably obvious that the BSU had evolved into a quiescent retirement home for a group of loyal long-term residents. Even an astute observer who strongly supported the unit (Sparks, 2002) recorded that:

> By the time I came there the unit collectively was a tired place . . . With rare exceptions, such as my interview, the community meeting was no longer the crucible of ideological debate and crackling personal tensions that it reputedly once had been. There was little left either of the ferment of artistic creativity purportedly associated with the unit's heyday in the 1970s (p. 567).

The same observer pointed out that:

> Some on both sides knew that the external perception was of a growing sense of marking time, of standing still, even of 'stagnation' within the unit community.

Both its prestige, as a place of innovation, experiment and transformation, and its pragmatic utility to Prison Service tacticians were in steep decline (p. 571).

The Scottish Prison Service, in 1993, set up a Working Party to review and seriously reconsider the status of the BSU. In its report, the Working Party (1994) observed that:

The near universal view is that in the absence of an active and continuously developing community, the BSU has become stagnant and fossilised. Many of the current prisoners have spent lengthy periods of time (in one case, 10 years) in the Unit, often actively refusing to move to another establishment, as this has been seen as a backward move, entailing too many sacrifices.

(Working Party, 1994, p. 17)

The report also noted that:

Only one of the current group of prisoners is regularly engaged in any kind of constructive activity and this is an activity from which he gains a significant financial profit. The remainder of the prisoners spend the majority of their time entertaining visitors, reading, watching television or sleeping (p. 18).

The 'bottom line' for the Working Group was the conclusion that:

The BSU is not [now] a model community and it is doubtful whether the current regime produces re-socialised, responsible prisoners who are ready and able to return to the mainstream. As such, the collusion which has perpetuated certain elements of the BSU mythology should not be allowed to continue' (*ibid.*).

One way of translating this assertion is that meaningful humane confinement must remain meaningful as well as humane. We must welcome any ameliorations of confinement, but cannot afford to tolerate the erosion of therapeutic principles and goals.

In other words, a humane setting must remain true to its mission. Ideally, such a setting should be able to consistently support the personal development of its residents; and ought to provide the sort of ambience that allows these residents to evolve and rehearse incipient pro-social dispositions and skills. As a precondition, of course, a humane prison setting has to try to survive, but the real point of the endeavour must be to demonstrate that it can effectively contribute to the common good.

References

Barker E (1980) The Penetanguishene program: A personal review. In: H Toch (ed) *Therapeutic Communities in Corrections.* Praeger, New York.

Commons WH (1940) Official Manual of the State Prison Colony. In: CR Doering (ed) *A Report on the Development of Penological Treatment at Norfolk Prison Colony in Massachusetts.* Bureau of Social Hygiene, New York.

Kennedy L (1982) Foreword. In: C Carrell and J Laing (eds) *The Special Unit BarlinniePrison: its evolution through its art.* Third Eye Centre, Glasgow.

Rothman DJ (2002) *Conscience and Convenience: the asylum and its alternatives in progressive America* (2e). Aldine De Gruyter, New York.

Scharf P (1980) Democracy and justice in a prison therapeutic community. In: H Toch (ed) *Therapeutic Communities in Corrections.* Praeger, New York.

Serrill MS (1982) Norfolk: A retrospective. New debate over a famous prison experiment. *Corrections Magazine.* **August**: 25–32.

Sparks R (2002) Out of the 'digger': The warrior's honour and the guilty observer. *Ethnography.* **3**(4): 556–81.

Studt E, Messinger SL and Wilson TP (1968) *C-Unit: search for community in prison.* Russell Sage Foundation, New York.

Working Party on Barlinnie Special Unit (1994) *Report: small units in the Scottish Prison Service.* Scottish Prison Service, Edinburgh.

Yahkub T (1940) A history of the state prison colony. In: CR Doering (ed) *A Report on the Development of Penological Treatment at Norfolk Prison Colony in Massachusetts.* Bureau of Social Hygiene, New York.

Chapter 2

First impressions

Kathy Page

Those who work inside the penal system perhaps inevitably become habituated to the extraordinary conditions, bizarre relationships and intense emotional atmosphere that make up their daily environment; it may be useful, then, to begin with an outsider's view.

Nottingham Prison is an archetype: a grim, brick-built, Victorian building featuring a gatehouse with a portcullis, surrounded by huge walls topped with razor wire and situated bang in the middle of a residential district. It is very like Wandsworth, outside which my parents would occasionally park the car on the way home from a visit to my grandmother. *That's where they put them*, they would tell me, whether to warn or reassure I can't be sure, *that's where they lock up men who do bad things.*

I fill out papers, hand over my bag, and follow a whistling officer through a series of locked doors and gates, across a courtyard decorated with orderly plantings of tulips and into an administrative wing painted apricot white. It's a group interview and once assembled we set off for a whistlestop tour: the dim, echoing wing, bathed in a stultifying silence punctuated by shouts and the echo of someone's radio; a cell complete with the bulge on the wall where once the treadmill was set; the tiny library; the slow-motion workshops; the education department humming in its fluorescent glare. We return to Administration, noting its relatively refreshing smells of paint, coffee and air freshener, and settle down to a dainty buffet prepared by inmates: vol au vents, quiche, celery sticks, radish flowers. One of the other candidates is an ex-prisoner, wearing a pinstripe suit and a fob watch, who arrived late and seems to me to be drunk. Another is an ultra-feminine woman with lashings of luxuriant hair.

One of the panel, a man with a tight collar and a lost-seeming face, leans forwards, asks:

'Why would a woman want to spend half her working week inside a male prison?'

A good question.

'To know what it is like?' I reply.

Later, on the train back to Norwich, I think about curiosity – about how, as a fiction writer, I spend much of my time imagining my way into other people's lives. Why? Isn't one life enough to keep me busy? Suppose I put all that effort into something 'real'? My mind runs to stories: Adam and Eve, Bluebeard, Cupid and Psyche – all of them about women who defy a prohibition against knowledge. The last two are especially interesting: Bluebeard's wife finds her way into her husband's bloody chamber and all but perishes there; Psyche wants to know who her invisible lover really is. Both stories tell of women making discoveries about the nature of men; both have been elaborately analysed by literary scholars and psychoanalysts alike, but at its most basic their message seems to be that curiosity frequently brings a woman far more than she bargained for.

When the job offer comes, I have to choose between it and a place on a prestigious scriptwriting course which I applied for earlier in the year. I feel I know what going back to school will be like. Curiosity prevails, and a few months later I return to Nottingham. My official title is Writer in Residence.

'Don't give an inch. Don't believe what they tell you. Remember, there's a reason why people are in here,' says the cheery-faced officer who takes me around on my walkabouts. 'You'll learn,' he says. I soon realise that all newcomers are constantly told by inmates and officers alike that they'll soon learn. I think that the meaning of this is: *you'll learn that the 'other side' are subhuman* and also: *you'll learn how to cope.*

The wing, painted in shades of grey, smells of stale food, dirty laundry and blocked toilets. A little natural light filters in from above, but it's a dim and colourless space, sometimes stultifyingly silent but often filled with a cacophony of yelling, banging and music of various types played simultaneously and loud. When men are on the move from one place to another the aggression is palpable. Everyone is watching everyone else and watching his own back at the same time. A swift blow, and before you know it two men are in a scrum on the floor, a whistle blows and six officers arrive.

'The first thing you have to do is to learn how to hate. To survive, that's what you must do,' says one of the first inmates I talk to. 'You hate *them*,' he explains, his voice rising, 'because of what they do to you and what they think of you. *They* hate *you* because of what you've done to get here, because they know you hate them and because you make them hate themselves . . . They've chosen, we haven't. And if the place goes up, *you'd* be one of *them*. I'm just telling you. That's how it is.' Veins stand out on his forehead and arms. 'Sorry. It's the fucking situation,' he concludes abruptly with a handshake and a nod, before walking off without giving any opportunity for a reply.

On the way from one building to another I meet a man wearing enormous, udder-like red rubber gloves and pushing a wheelbarrow. His job is to pick up the excrement thrown from cell windows during the night.

'Writing? I'm afraid to say,' he tells me screwing his eyes up against the sun, 'that whatever you think you're here for, you'll just be wanking material.'

In the solitary block a hollow-cheeked man gestures at a newly installed stainless steel sink and toilet in his cell, one of the sanitary units which will eventually put an end to slopping out. Heavily bolted to the floor, gleaming, it dominates the small room like an altar. He is, he tells me in a quiet monotonous voice, one of the lucky ones.

'Of course, I'd rather not slop out. But look at it this way: you could be slopping out in another situation – say it was a hospital in wartime or a monastery or something' – he smiles suddenly as if the place has appeared to him, benevolently transformed – 'it wouldn't bother you. What matters is the rest of it, what goes on. They've changed the symbol, but what it was meaning is still there.' He pauses, points at the unit, 'It says *you're shit.*' I look around the cell, take in the cardboard furniture, the three oranges on the windowsill, the pile of books. What are they saying?

'I don't decorate,' he says. 'Why pretend. It's not a home.'

'Had enough for now?' the officer asks a while later. Well, yes – and I'm thinking that a constant stream of these kinds of encounters is going to take its toll.

'You just block it out,' the officer tells me. 'Like I said, they've done something wrong and that's why they're here.' But aren't they here to be rehabilitated? Wasn't there a notice to that effect over the door as I came in? I can't help feeling that's going to be an uphill task in a place where everyone seems at loggerheads and ready to erupt.

'Well,' he says, 'you read the files, that's what I advise.'

In Education, they disagree. They mostly don't read the files. They find it gets in the way of relating to the person as he is now; they want to build on the good, not hark back to the bad. Education, sited in a flimsy portakabin in the main courtyard, is almost entirely staffed by women. Literacy, numeracy, sociology, cooking – and now creative writing – are delivered along with proper tea and chocolate biscuits. There are copies of the *Guardian* and the *Times* to borrow, computers to use. The buildings are cramped, drab and utterly airless, and attending classes means relegation to a minimum wage but nonetheless there is always a waiting list for Education. It is an oasis of purposefulness in a place where, collectively, millennia of time must be wasted. It is also a place where men go to hear female voices, have interesting conversations, smell perfume, see the carefully chosen, modest but colourful clothes, and imagine what is beneath them. As in any workplace, or perhaps even more so, attractions and relationships form. One of the staff, I learn, is engaged to marry a former inmate; she's not the first and won't be the last. Education holds out the possibility of intimacy, or at least the means to it.

In the wider prison, most of the time spoken language is of little use. People blot out the words and read the body. They gesture: draw a line across the throat, give the finger, push their chair back so it screams on the floor, then add a few expletives for emphasis. But in Education it seems that people do at least sometimes use language for more complex communication, to connect with the other person rather than push them away. Outside the computer room I meet a muscular, much scarred man with a shaved head who is waiting for his turn. He begins with a litany of the system's deficiencies and injustices, but then brightens and tells me:

'One good very good thing, though. Being here has improved my marriage one hundred per cent.' The impossibility of violence is definitely part of it, he admits, but what's really got him going is the letter-writing. He's writing his wife long, introspective letters, opening up to her in just the way women are always saying they want men to do. He didn't have time for all that before. And he's reading what she writes back, getting to know her. Ten years together and he didn't know her at all before, he says. She was just a cartoon figure in his head, with *woman* written underneath . . .

I have to say that's often how I feel here. It's not a place where you can forget your gender. Cat calls and banter apart, I'm acutely aware of the difference between me and the inmates and the officers alike (I feel too that they are more like each other than either would ever admit). It's hard living in 'their' world. I work differently and this difference is wanted and despised at the same time, just as it is outside, but with even greater intensity. This is not simply about anatomy and the roles we take on; it seems to be about what kind of communication is possible, and a huge, barely acknowledged need for contact. There is an expectation that I, as one of the women, will listen sympathetically, but not challenge. Sometimes an answer of any kind is unwelcome; every encounter has its own difficult dynamics and, indeed, silence is often the best way to proceed.

Not long ago, a man came up to me in wing corridor and offered his hand to shake. He gripped mine as if to kill it.

'Still here?' he asked, standing in a doorway, half in, half out. 'When I last saw you' – I remembered it was at the gate, a battered car delivering him back to the prison, his mates returning him and his suitcase in a cloud of smoke from a week's home leave – 'when I last saw you, I was well outta my head.' He paused. His hips were as thin as a child's, his skin pricked with fresh prison blue tattoos.

'I'm out again this Friday. My old lady died, see. So they have to let me out. I knew her seventeen years.' As soon as I drew breath to speak, he ground the butt of his cigarette under his heel and said, 'So long. See you.' A week later, I saw the same man again, wandering around with his eyes scoured bloody red from an accident with the strimmer. He said he was going to sue the Home Office.

'Him?' a fellow prisoner scoffed. 'Me, I don't talk. I *do*. All talk. Mouth. Blather. *Words.*'

Often it's the act of speaking which provides release, rather than what has been said. The day's talk is a series of outbursts, witnessed by another person or persons, who block most of it out. Sentences don't rate finishing. Details are immaterial. One stupid cunt is much like another. '*See? See?*' a man will ask, but he won't believe you if you say yes. Stories are left unfinished. 'End of Story' stands in for the crisis point of an account; the rest – the culminating violence and its aftermath, feeling, meaning – these are passed right over. Inevitable, perhaps, or uninteresting: 'So then he came up to me. *End of Story.*' As if all stories were the same and ended that way.

The officers' equivalent is a shrug.

'How are you?' I ask the key man on my way out.

'What can you expect?' he replies. 'Years since I did anything constructive.' He holds my gaze as he opens the outer gate. 'Don't,' he adds quietly, '*Don't* tell me I can always get out. I need the money and that's that.' At this, another officer emerges from the gatehouse. He's virtually dancing on the spot, his face red; his eyes glitter with aggressive jocularity.

'He's just having you on! He loves it really. It's the uniform, see.' The laughter that follows this is like machine-gun fire, and then the door slams shut.

I find the constant hostility almost unbearable. Speakers walk away from each other, teachers, me, mid-sentence. No one can see any point in trying to sort out a misunderstanding. Explanations are pointless. Most of what was said is, or is seen as, lies. What writers do in life, the passion to return again and again to words, checking out that what they say is what was meant, listening to how they sound, arranging them in the best possible order – in the prison, all that is tantamount to madness. To want language to work, to reach another person, is to want both myself and the other person to matter. To admit hope. And that of course lays you open. Forget it! *End of.*

A group of six turn up for the first writing workshop, held in Education's murky portakabin.

'Would you read this out for me?' one of them asks. 'I don't want my voice to shake.' Everyone in the room understands the emergency; the unspoken rule seems to be that a man must squeeze his hurts very small and, if they don't disappear, let them explode straight out into rage; eventually the accumulation of anger will create a fury sufficient to blot out even the first tremors of other feelings and be there, a weapon against everything, ready at his fingertips . . . But he's lost his grip, and so I oblige, and read the two paragraphs aloud. They describe a typical childhood beating: an eight-year-old's terror, trapped in the over-furnished front room of a railway terrace, hearing the carriage clock tick and watching as his father unbuckled his belt and slowly extracted it from the loops of his waistband.

'I wrote something too,' another man says, and reads, for himself, an account of being woken in the middle of the night by his alcoholic mother, made to complete the day's chores, and then, as a punishment, sent to sleep in the bathtub.

And so, all of a sudden, I find myself the completely untrained facilitator of a kind of what seems to want to be a therapy, as much as a writing, group. Somehow I've got to steer a manageable course, to give the content some of the attention it's due, without getting us out of all our depths . . . It's an unenviable role, but we are at least talking, and listening, almost as if we were somewhere else.

I don't know what I expected, but it wasn't this.

I'm aware that inmates who feel they have told you too much often cut you dead the next time they see you, so it is quite possible that even after this no one, or else a completely different set of people, will turn up next week. On the other hand, it might just work. We could get used to this material and then, eventually, we might ask ourselves what purpose, public or private, it might serve to present it in words? We might even, eventually, I fantasise, discuss structure and the use of active verbs . . .

Over time, the writing becomes less straightforwardly autobiographical and psychologically more complex. A story, for instance, about three triplets in the womb which the writer calls 'that dark, loving place'. 'It wasn't a battle of wills,' he writes 'but of needs and wants.' The female foetus takes more than her share of sustenance and when the narrator's brother dies before term, 'she no longer needed to steal it, she simply claimed it as her own'. One of the teachers is pregnant and brings in the printout of a recent ultrasound scan. Another inmate makes an ink drawing of the three foetuses, floating in black.

I'm presented with all kinds of narratives: elaborate science fiction and fantasy, hugely ambitious thrillers, ghost stories, even Mills and Boon-type romances. I find the stories about family the most compelling, partly for what they suggest about the writer's past, but also because they seem to connect with the prison itself. No one here calls the prison a family because, notwithstanding the experiences many here have had, a family is after all supposed to be a good place; nonetheless, it strikes me that it does have the shape of one. I would say the prison is the kind of family where the men set the rules and the women, doing their best to be kind, sometimes break them but may also threaten, when desperate: 'Wait 'til your father gets home.' It's the kind of family where the children fight each other for what scraps of attention and affection are available, where real communication is minimal and self-expression oblique. People cry in secret and everyone suffers.

I have been given my own keys, and walk through the wing during evening association. There's the usual din of radios and shouting. Light flickers over taut pale faces as the men sit in rows to watch a documentary about a massacre in Vietnam. Roll-ups are passed from hand to hand, grabbed, fought over; the smoke of these thin cigarettes made from butt ends smells like death itself. Just outside the TV room, there's a man with a bleeding head, ignored by others who pass by. Men with tiny pupils and frozen faces lean against the walls, just staring out. A considerable number of cells are still locked, because their inhabitants prefer not to associate. Soon, I'm told, there will be a TV set in every cell. Along with installation of sanitation, this is supposed to signify a more humane approach but, like the man I met on day one, I'm not convinced. It's the way people relate to each other that seems to be the problem. How can you change that? Is anyone trying?

'Eventually, you'll see the truth,' intones the officer I chat with on my way out, and I think, frivolously, of some exotic butterfly fluttering in the immense dim space of B wing and me running hopelessly after it with a net. All the same, I think, it is probably is time I read some files.

The files have to be read in the room in which they are kept and I spend most of a day there. I learn in detail of the physical agonies and mental torture, the trail of suffering that men I have come to know as thoughtful, helpful types and also, in some cases, as neglected or abused children, have left behind them. I learn that I can be at the same time overwhelmed with pity for and repelled by the actions of the very same person. He is both vulnerable and cruel.

Why would a woman want to spend half her working week inside a men's prison? Why indeed.

The place presses down on me, a heavy weight. I won't get used to it, thank God, but I've got to get through the year. I want to do something that transforms the prison, even momentarily. Reading the script of *Our Country's Good* (Wertenbaker, 1991) makes me think that perhaps we too could stage a play. Something that many people can have a part in; a comedy of some kind. We could write it in the workshop. The Governor, to the collective surprise of the education department, does not say no, and so I find myself sitting in a cubby hole in education, touting for people to join the newly formed improvisation and drama group. We are going to learn acting and write the play at the same time. We'll have a script by the end of September, and three months to rehearse it.

I sign a few up, but there is a powerfully built black man with a mono-tonous, hoarse voice who doesn't want to put his name down but won't go away either. *It just won't work*, he tells me, shaking his head from side to side. *No way*, he says, following me into the corridor, stooped, shaking his head from side to side. *No way, no way, it won't ever work.*

He could, of course, be right. I've not done anything even remotely like this before, and I'm getting it all from books. So, suppose I tell them to exhale slowly, making an *aaaaah* sound and letting their voice come from their solar plexus – will they do it? Will they wander blindfolded around the room with only their hands to guide them?

On the day of the first session, I find my hoarse ghost, hovering at the door of the room we have been assigned.

'Do you want to join us?'

'No way . . . I just came to watch.'

There's nothing for it but to shut the door and begin. We jump and yell and then tiptoe about. We move onto nonsense chants and other people's walks. Soon we have a room full of women in high heels, and then a room full of two-year-olds. Then babies, lying on their backs. Teenagers. Drunks.

Months later, we are using the same room as a make-up and dressing room. We have overcome the ghosting of several of the actors, the tantrums thrown by others. With the help of local art school students we have managed to make scenery without using scissors ourselves and we have proper, raised seating lent by the County Council. The chaplain has reluctantly allowed us to use the chapel for the performances, even though he disapproves of the profane content of our play, a pantomime loosely based on Cinderella. Half the cast are in drag; the good fairy is a huge, tattooed body builder with a shaved head who wears a tutu, fishnet tights and Dr Marten's boots. The men are quieter than usual as they check their costumes and have their greasepaint applied; their eyes glitter with a blend of apprehension and excitement. On our way to the chapel we all stop, rooted to the spot by the sight and sounds of a long crocodile of junior school children crossing the barren courtyard.

I watch from behind the set, ready to nudge onto stage anyone who becomes mesmerised by the action and forgets that he's part of it too. The music comes on cue; the kids titter, giggle, then roar with laughter and scream the familiar refrains:

'Oh, yes we ARE!'

'He's BEHIND you!!'

The play is performed for children, VIPs and inmates only, and, naturally, the jokes are different every time. Afterwards, letters of thanks flood in and we feel we've done something that broke the spell of the place: we worked as a kind of team, and we connected to the world outside. For a time at least, we were somewhere else.

In January, I look in the mirror and realise that over the past nine months my haircut has by increments become shorter and more severe; that there's a sallow look to my skin and deep purple shading under my eyes. What next, tattoos? Still, there are only a few more months to go. I can't wait to leave . . . When at last I do so, exiting with my holdall of books and tapes after a farewell buffet-cum-book launch for the Writing Group's anthology, I know that the place and the people and the problem: *how do we deal with people who have hurt us?* will haunt me for years to come.

I worked in HMP Nottingham for a year from 1991–2. At the time it was a Category B men's prison with something of a reputation as a dumping ground for difficult men. Writer's residencies are an arrangement whereby a writer is attached half-time to an institution with a brief to develop the writing skills of those within it; less clearly stated but nonetheless implicit is the idea that the writer will in some way learn from and may be inspired to write about his or her experience of the institution. A classic account in this tradition is *Inside Time* by Ken Smith, (Smith, 1989) one of the first Writers in Residence, who worked from 1985–6 in Wormwood Scrubs. As well as an anthology of inmates' writing (Page, 1992), a novel of mine, *Alphabet* (Page, 2004), eventually arose out of my year in Nottingham; what you have read here is a personal account culled from notes I made at the time.

References

Page K (ed) (1992) *Temporary Release: an anthology of inmates' writings*. Nottingham County Council, Nottingham.
Page K (2004) *Alphabet*. Weidenfeld & Nicolson, London.
Smith K (1989) *Inside Time*. Harrap, London.
Wertenbaker T (1991) *Our Country's Good*. Methuen, London.

Chapter 3

Life inside

Erwin James

There was no doubt about the purpose of imprisonment in my case. My crimes had been so serious that there had been no alternative but that I should be separated from society for a long time. When he sentenced me, the judge who presided over my trial made no comments regarding how he expected me to spend my time in prison. Neither did he comment on what society would be expecting of me during my incarceration. His job was simply to pass sentence. I received mandatory life.

Before then I'd had only a modest degree of experience of prison custody. At the age of 17, I served six months in a detention centre (the so-called 'short, sharp shock' treatment, popular with politicians in the 1970s). When I was 18, I spent 13 months undergoing Borstal training, and at 23, I spent six weeks in a London 'local' prison for breaching a community service order. But these earlier custodial experiences gave me no sense of what life was going to be like as a long-term prisoner in the adult system. As far as I could tell throughout all of these periods of being locked up, the only real aim among my fellow prisoners and I was to do the time and get released.

In the detention centre it seemed that the purpose of the prison officers was to subject the 'trainees' as we were termed, to a rigorous regime of unrelenting 'discipline' which often included violence. The idea, I guess, was to shock us so that we would be deterred from coming back for more, and go on to into lead law-abiding lives. Whenever we moved around the institution, to work or to the refectory, we had to march quickly. Officers never spoke to us in normal tones, only shouted or gave us 'orders' with voices raised.

The physical education officers were particularly enthusiastic about dishing out physical punishment. Like many of the youngsters serving time in the institution, I had experienced violence and intimidation from adults from an early age and so was not especially perturbed by this behaviour. In one incident during a physical education session, the track-suited officer in charge instructed a group of us to crouch down in a line behind him and place our hands on the hips of the person in front of us. I happened to be situated immediately behind the officer. As my hands touched him the officer sprang to his full height and screamed, 'Are you fucking queer? Do you fancy me?' before launching a punch which landed across the side of my head. In spite of being stunned I managed to say, 'No, sir.' The officer then screamed a stream of expletives at me concluding with, 'Why? What's fucking wrong with me?' before hitting me across the head again. Clearly the purpose of his actions was to terrorise the group. But the fact that I barely flinched as the officer's blows landed brought me a large measure of respect from my fellow trainees. Being perceived as 'hard' was something most of us aspired to. However hard we were thought to be by our peers determined the place we were allocated on the trainee hierarchy.

When I was released from detention centre I was fitter than at any other time of my life. I prided myself on being 'tough' and resilient to whatever life had in store for me. Unfortunately I returned to an unsettled lifestyle, with the problems which had contributed to my earlier antisocial behaviour and subsequent criminal convictions no nearer to being resolved, but now tougher on the outside. Within months I was back in custody, this time in a 'closed' Borstal.[1] Borstal training was different to life in the detention centre. In particular, there was more emphasis on teaching trainees work skills and there was more 'association' time (time spent in open conditions with other prisoners). I undertook a welding course and got involved in sports activities. There were also evening classes, where arts and crafts were taught.

Though the regime of the institution did not countenance fear and intimidation from the prison officers, there still existed a firmly established prison culture hierarchy which strictly divided the prisoners and the staff. 'Grassing', giving information about fellow prisoners to the authorities, was treated as the most serious breach of the prisoners' 'code' and would be met with commensurately serious violence if discovered. The hierarchy was also more sharply defined. As well as perceived toughness, the offence that a prisoner had been convicted of was very relevant to his place in the pecking order. Sex offenders were on the lowest end of the scale. Armed robbers, especially those who had committed crimes using firearms, were at the top end. We were all vulnerable, but most of us acted towards each other with exaggerated bravado and machismo. Fights in the association room away from the eyes of the supervising prison officers were regular occurrences, as were ambushes of suspected sex offenders or grasses in the bath-house. We were prisoners, all of us criminals convicted of an array of relatively serious offences, but the main thing we had in common was that we were emotionally immature adolescent boys, some of whom were more socially inadequate than others. The more vulnerable and needy among us suffered the most.

After Borstal I returned once again to a directionless way of life. The welding I'd learned gave me more scope for obtaining work. But without a settled home life and the ability to focus on building a regular future I was soon back committing criminal offences. The offences escalated in seriousness. I received a community service order after being convicted of assault occasioning actual bodily harm, but then failed to complete the community work and as a result I was committed to prison for six weeks. The majority of this time inside was spent locked in a cell with two other prisoners for 22 hours a day, being let out only for an hour's exercise in the prison yard and to collect our food at meal times and empty our toilet buckets. I spent most of the time during those six weeks sleeping. This appeared to be the way of things for short-term prisoners in local prisons.

Throughout these comparatively short periods of prison time I never considered whether the institutions I was held in were humane institutions or otherwise. For one, my education level was quite low, having received a limited formal education beforehand. I had never been someone who thought about social policies or issues. The lifestyle I led meant that I existed on the fringes of mainstream society. Most of the offences I committed were acquisitive or involved low levels of violence, such as criminal damage or common assault. I'd never considered the purpose of incarceration other than as a punishment for my bad behaviour. Since the age of 10, when I'd been taken into the care system, I'd thought of myself as a criminal. If I got caught committing criminal offences I expected to go to court and receive punishment. If the punishment involved a period of imprisonment I accepted whatever that entailed without a moment's analysis.

When I received my life sentence my attitude was pretty much the same. I understood the seriousness of my situation, but in an odd way I was glad of the life sentence as it meant that the life I had led before, which had brought so much unhappiness and distress to so many people, including myself, was over. My relief, however, was short-lived. The memory of my first day as a life sentenced prisoner is still vivid. First I'm taken from court to a 'local' prison where I will remain until I'm allocated to a long-term prison. Once 'processed' I'm directed to the centre of the prison and sent onto the long-termers wing, one of six wings holding around 200 prisoners each that stretch out from the centre. I walk along a gantry-style landing about a metre wide. Wire mesh stretches across the landings to stop people plunging over the safety rail, either by choice or at the point of force from someone else. I'm on the third floor – 'the threes'. I'm carrying a plastic bucket inside which clatters a plastic cup, knife, fork and spoon. Under my arm I have a 'bedroll': two flannel sheets rolled up inside two coarse blankets.

I'm guided to my cell by a large prison officer sporting a handlebar moustache. The peak of his cap has been 'slashed' so it fits low over the bridge of his nose. We reach my allocated cell and with a noisy rattle of his keys he unlocks the door and pushes it open. He's smiling: 'In you go, son, don't be shy.' The door slams shut behind me. The cell is dimly lit by a small, grime-covered fluorescent light. The walls are covered in cracked and flaking emulsion. There's a table, a chair, and a metal bed with a stained mattress and half a foam pillow. The heavily barred window high up on the wall is closed, and the urine-tainted air makes me want to retch. I sit down on the bed. Time to collect my thoughts – but no, I hear a sound like rolling thunder approaching fast, and suddenly the cell door is unlocked and pushed open again. 'Slop out and get your evening meal,' instructs handlebars.

A stream of denim-clad men in identical blue-and-white-striped shirts are shuffling past my door. I step out and join the flux. Down two flights of metal stairs to the ground floor; we're headed towards a set of trestle tables. A row of prisoners in white are serving food. Before I get there I am stopped in my tracks by a scream: 'He's fuckin' dead meat! Nonce! He's fuckin' dead meat!' I turn and see two men: one wields a mop handle, the other a metal bucket. They are using the domestic implements to beat a third prisoner who cowers in a cell doorway. 'He's fuckin' dead meat!'

Suddenly I'm aware that no one else is stopping. Nobody is intervening. Few even look in the direction of the violence. I fall back in line, pick up a tray, collect my meal and return to my cell. As I sit on the chair and spoon down the food, all thoughts and feelings about why I am in prison are relegated. My first priority, I now understand, is to learn to survive.

The idea of prison as a place to be survived was exacerbated when during my first Christmas inside the man in the cell directly above mine hanged himself from the bars of his cell window with a cord made from braided strips of bed sheet. I'd heard sounds in the early hours: footsteps, jangling keys, hushed voices. I rolled over and went back to sleep. Only in the Christmas morning breakfast queue did I learn what had happened. The mood of the queue was sombre, but still people joked. Someone ducked and shouted, 'One off on the fours, sir!' (This was a parody of how officers would relay the information to their colleagues in the control room whenever for any reason a prisoner moved from the wing to another part of the prison.) Somebody else asked for more cereals (in those days cereals were only ever served on public holidays). 'What do mean there ain't none spare? I'll have his,' he said, pointing up to the fours landing. Some of us laughed, but all of us kept our true thoughts about what had happened to ourselves. Self-inflicted death in prison, I was to learn, was something I was going to have to get used to.

My first year was spent on what is commonly termed 23-hour bang-up. During that time there were two more self-inflicted deaths in the jail. I did not know any of the people who had taken their own lives, and though my initial reaction on hearing the news was a deep internal shiver, like almost everyone else, I did not dwell for too long on their plight. The days passed with numbing monotony, all were much the same as the first, punctuated only by the doors opening for slop out and food, and an hour's exercise if the weather was not 'inclement'. The regime was not dissimilar from the six weeks I'd done for breaching the community service order some years earlier, except without the sleeping. I knew I had years like this ahead of me and I understood that to survive it I'd have to stay awake and learn. I spent a lot of time reading, exercising and thinking. I realised quickly that even though I felt secure for the first time for as long as I could remember, there was also a frightening precariousness to prison life. Though the cell doors were only opened briefly at the designated times, it was long enough for incidents of violence to take place. This violence was usually the result of arguments that had started during the shouting out of cell windows, or, just like in the Borstal, it involved ambushes of suspected sex offenders or attacks on former acquaintances who had turned informer. Just like in Borstal, the 'nonces' and 'grasses' were the whipping boys on a prison wing. But violent incidents could also occur spontaneously. Bumping into someone on the landing, catching the eye of someone who didn't appreciate being 'looked at' or simply appearing obviously vulnerable could be enough to unleash the pent-up frustration generated by the long periods of confinement.

The hierarchy was important. Looking like you could handle yourself in a fight ensured a certain amount of respect. This was why I embarked on a rigorous in-cell fitness routine of press-ups, sit-ups and running on the spot every day without fail until I was drenched in sweat. Within a few weeks I had established a disciplined way of living that was almost ritualised: sleep, eat, read, exercise, wash, eat, read, sleep. As the time went on, however, I learned that it might be possible to benefit from the prison experience.

After the year spent on bang-up I was transferred to a high-security long-term prison. Here, the time we spent locked in our cells was around 14 hours out of 24. It was a very different set up to what I'd previously experienced. The day-to-day regime included time spent working, in workshops (metal fabrication, or manufacturing prison clothing), cleaning, or for a maximum of ten per cent of the prison population, attending education classes. We were also allowed to use the gym a couple of times a week and go out on the exercise yard every day. It was a much better regime than the one I'd left behind. But that didn't stop people taking their own lives. The week before my arrival a man serving a life sentence had committed suicide by jumping from the top landing onto the 'centre' – the hexagonal area where the four wings of the prison merged and from where the prison population was observed and controlled. It was the only area that had no protective meshing to break the cavernous space. The spectacular manner of this man's passing was a constant topic of conversation on the landings, very little of which was sympathetic. He was christened 'Superman'. I found out that his action had followed a call to his wing office where he had been told that his case for release would not be considered for at least another thirteen years (in prisoner jargon he'd received a 'thirteen-year knockback'). He had served four years, which, because of the way the system worked in those days, meant that he would have to serve at least 20 years in total. It was believed that release was normally granted three years after the end of the knockback period. I was learning fast that unexpected death in prison was a regular occurrence. In that prison especially, it had lost its power to shock. In the preceding four years, as well as the average number of apparent suicides, there had been three prisoner-on-prisoner killings.

A couple of weeks or so after my arrival a wing governor called me to his office. He was a pleasant man, whose purpose for this meeting, I guessed, was to assess my mental and psychological state. He asked me about my sentence, about how I felt I was coping. Then he said something totally unexpected. 'My job,' he said, looking me firmly in the eye, 'is to get you back out there and functioning properly.' The governor's words rang in my head for days. But it was clear that there was some conflict in attitudes among prison staff. The prison officers had a very similar attitude to those I had encountered in the last prison. They made it clear that this was their environment, their prison, and that I was very much under their control. It was clear to me that above all they considered the main purpose of their job was to keep me in, regardless of how I functioned. I wasn't sure if there was any official understanding that they would make any type of contribution to my personal development.

Within a few months of my arrival at the long-term prison I came to the conclusion that the prison structure – the prison officer hierarchy, buildings, fabric and regime – was a long-established hostile entity which had the effect of systematically undermining any sense of a shared humanity among its inhabitants. In this respect there was little difference between it and the previous so-called local establishment. As time went on this sense of dehumanisation became more apparent. That is not to say that we, the prisoners, did not think of ourselves as human. But the feeling that the system whose mercy we were at resented us – despised us, in fact – created a deep psychological detachment. Newspapers provided us with society's general view of prisons and prisoners, and since the majority of newspapers were popular tabloids which depicted prisoners almost as a different species of creature to the 'law-abiding majority' the effect was to reinforce the feeling of detachment. In spite of this, there was little sense of commonality among us. Like my neighbours I perceived my fellow prisoners as the greatest source of potential harm in the prison. I believe that this was why there was so much paranoia and such a high level of social imbalance amongst those of us serving the longest sentences. People who had entered prison with mental health problems fared the least well.

And yet, for all the negativity of life on the wing, there were elements of the prison regime that provided great benefit to prisoners. For me the most important was the lively education department. In my own case my earlier limited formal education and life experiences had led me to believe that any further education would have little if any positive impact. My feelings about myself were such that I did not believe myself to be capable of being educated any further.

One day I was summoned for an interview with the wing psychologist. I was made aware of the 'call up' when I arrived back on the wing from the morning session in the workshop to see my name chalked on the wing noticeboard, followed by the words: 'Psycho call up.' It was the same for anyone who needed to be seen by the psychologist, and both prison staff and prisoners thought it was funny. The psychologist's name was Joan Branton. Ms Branton's approach was to gradually get to know the people on the wing she had to assess and write about through a series of such call ups. In my case these were to take place over a period of around two years.

Our exchanges took the form of hour-long conversations during which Ms Branton would gently probe my past and explore my life history up to the point of my life imprisonment. Her sensitive manner helped to create trust between us, so much so that I considered this relationship to be the first major positive influence in my life. Ms Branton's guidance and encouragement were crucial in determining the path the rest of my time in prison followed.

'You must get an education,' she implored. 'You are capable and very able. You owe it to yourself to use this time in the most constructive way possible.' This was the general conclusion to most of our early conversations until finally I was persuaded that I might indeed have some potential. The most difficult aspect of our meetings was having to pick apart the criminal actions that had led to my life sentence. These were explored to exhaustion in the minutest of detail. Yet she always ensured I left the office with something positive to focus on. Ms Branton was able to convince me that in spite of all that had happened, I was still valuable and could still become someone who could make a meaningful contribution to my community, whether that was inside or outside.

With Ms Branton's support I enrolled on evening classes in the education department. I took GCSEs in English, Maths and French, and passed all three within a year. With each achievement my sense of self-worth and self-belief was bolstered. I felt I owed it to Ms Branton to make the maximum effort to succeed. I also wanted the governor who said his job was to get me back out again to see that I was becoming someone he might one day be able to trust.

Thanks to Ms Branton's recommendation I was offered a job in the prison's Braille Transcription Unit. It was work that required mental discipline and consistency, totally unlike any work I had ever before undertaken. Though challenging, I found it incredibly satisfying and worthwhile. For the first time in my life I was making an effort to assist people who had a specific need that was greater than mine. The prison officer instructors had the opposite attitude to those who worked on the landings, the 'discipline' officers. The Braille Unit officers treated the 20 or so prisoners in the Unit with some respect and courtesy. They made us feel like workers – employees – first, and prisoners second. Eventually I was accepted to enrol on an Open University degree course. During the day I worked in the Braille Unit and undertook my degree course studies in my cell at night. I found that the constant use of my mind for work and study was the most liberating experience I'd ever had. In spite of my incarcerated state I felt that I was living with a purpose at last. It was ironic that this should occur in a high-security prison, but it is indicative of the dissatisfaction I'd felt with life before my imprisonment. I suddenly began to feel that I was making the kind of contribution to my community that I'd always been capable of, but had never had the appropriate circumstances in which to develop the skills necessary.

Another positive influence was the wing probation officer. The man's name was Brian Whately. Mr Whately made a point of greeting people when they returned from work at lunchtime or in the afternoon. He went out of his way to strike up conversations, sharing a little of his own life, news about his latest fishing trip or music interests. His polite and genuine interest in the wellbeing of the prisoners had an ameliorating effect on us. His manner, along with that of Ms Branton and the wing governor, was the most important source of humane contact. This was in stark contrast to the manner of the majority of the prison officers, who almost to a man spoke down to prisoners in a patronising and often intimidating manner. The few officers that demonstrated positive attitudes towards prisoners shone like beacons, but little of their respect or courtesy was genuinely reciprocated. For the prisoner, endeavouring to exist between the two conflicting attitudes made life uncertain, hence the detachment and the sense that we were living in ideological no-man's-land.

This to me became the paradox of prison life. On the one hand there were people who worked in the prison, and could be found in all prison worker positions, who saw their roles as life enhancers, guiders, encouragers, enablers. Such people represented the pockets of humanity in a prison. On the other hand there were those who worked there who saw prison as a strictly punitive experience and their role to facilitate a punitive atmosphere. Prison officers made up the majority of the latter. Whenever there were high-profile crimes in the news accompanied by headlines expressing outrage and disgust at the perpetrators, attitudes among many uniformed prison staff were noticeably affected. It seemed as if they took it upon themselves, almost as if it was their duty, to express a harsher attitude towards prisoners on behalf of 'the public'. The attitudes of most non-uniformed staff seemed unaffected by 'public outcry'. It was clear that the two groups represented a philosophical battle: the idea of 'rehabilitation' versus the idea of 'retribution'. It was clear also that this conflict was the main cause of stress for all who worked and lived in the prison community. As far as I could see, this conflict was responsible for the overall lack of an agreed collective purpose.

My view was that, though fellow prisoners could cause each other great discomfort and harm, fundamentally the majority wanted to use their time constructively. Most of us sought peace and change. Very few rejoiced in their role as prisoners, criminals. Those among us who appeared not to care were either mentally unhealthy or had psychological and behavioural difficulties that were too deeply rooted to be resolved without intense palliative care, which was unavailable in the mainstream prison environment. It felt like the system, for all the life-improving facilities that were available, was intrinsically loaded against anyone succeeding in making it work in a beneficial way. People who achieved, either in education or in acquiring work skills, or in any aspect of personal development, appeared to do so by overcoming the system's in-built destructiveness: unhelpful or obstructive prison staff; stifling bureaucracy; faceless decision-makers (inexplicable decisions); robust living conditions; failure to recognise behaviour that was symptomatic of poor mental health, etc. The overall feeling was that the system existed to feed itself and not to promote the wellbeing and future prospects of its prisoners. In spite of the occasional influence of a humane prison governor or prison officer, psychologist or probation officer, chaplain or teacher, the system just ground along, wearing people down on both sides of the divide.

As the years passed I became more and more determined not to succumb to the reductive and destructive effect of prison life. Each time I was transferred I found a prison community with a similar mix of personalities, amongst prisoners, and among staff. I stayed strong, in the gym and by running in the yard or around the sports field if there was one so that I would be able to seek out facilities and activities that would help me to strengthen my character. I was lucky in that I did not need too much encouragement and support to maintain my momentum. A little humanity went a long, long way. At the end of my 20 years I was left with the belief that the majority of people who go to prison would like to change, to become responsible, law-abiding adults. Since the same majority are those who need the maximum of encouragement, support and resources, it should not be surprising that the prison experience does not produce more successful results with regard to the reduction of reoffending after release. Even when people who go to prison do address their failings and make an effort to plan and prepare for a more satisfying and successful life outside, often the circumstances they find themselves in once back out there make it difficult, if not impossible, to achieve that dream. Unless there is the support of family and friends, and unless they have accommodation and work, no matter how motivated they might be, the odds are stacked against them. The fact that people often do succeed in leading crime-free lives in spite of the system is a testament to human resilience and resourcefulness. There were 1247 self-inflicted deaths among prisoners in prisons in England and Wales during the time I was serving my sentence. There were thousands more resuscitations by prison staff. It is only thanks to the adaptability of human beings, and their capacity to endure mental and physical discomfort, that the figures for both are not higher. While I remain grateful for what I gained from my prison experience, I'm left with the feeling that overall it was something that I survived, undoubtedly against the odds.

Note

1 Formerly used in Great Britain for delinquent boys aged 16 to 21. The idea originated (1895) with the Gladstone Committee as an attempt to reform young offenders. The first institution was established (1902) at Borstal Prison, Kent, England. Main elements in the Borstal programmes included education, regular work, character formation, discipline, obedience and respect for authority. Acts of violence in Borstal could result in a birching, which was the only official corporal punishment allowed. However, Borstal governors openly used canes and heavy leather straps long after birching had been stopped, but there were very few official complaints from lads who were more concerned with getting out than having extra time added to their sentence by trying to complain to unsympathetic authorities. The Criminal Justice Act 1982 abolished the Borstal system.

Chapter 4

Psychopathological considerations of prison systems

David Jones

Introduction

This chapter considers some of the powerful emotional forces that exert an effect in organisations. My contention is that the criminal justice system exists at the interface between, on the one hand, highly sensitive political and cultural forces and, on the other, the disturbed, aggressive world of prisoners, and is particularly prone to be influenced by the currents and eddies created by these conflicting forces. Since many of these forces are unconscious and most of the professional players are trained to respond to concrete situations in rapid time, the opportunity for reflective thinking of a kind that can moderate impulsive behaviour and plan a culture which is flexible and conducive to rehabilitation are limited.

Much of the reflective thinking in this area is conducted by academics and some of their contributions are contained in this volume. However, the actual beneficial effects of such contributions can be slow in arriving. For example, Kupers (*see* Chapter 5) provides a clarity of vision in relation to the common problem of mental illness induced and made worse through imprisonment, together with a recipe for its reversal. He does so from the position of a visiting expert whose influence may be through painstaking negotiation with senior management or after lengthy court procedures.

However, staff working on the floor of the prison block and the management levels just above this can achieve a most profound and positive influence through their everyday contact. But the work of maintaining standards and absorbing anxiety is usually counter-subcultural, attritional and difficult. It can seem intrusive and conflictual and may threaten senior prison managers who can sometimes view themselves rather like a sea captain or army general. For inexperienced and anxious junior staff, and senior managers worried about losing their 'ship' and their job, working with disturbed prisoners can in any case be emotionally depleting and frustrating.

Using the example of a highly dramatic series of events in a prison with an international reputation for its humane regime I consider the unconscious dynamics that operate in this field. It is an account of these incidents mainly from a psychoanalytic perspective put in straightforward terms. But it can only represent at best several tessarae in a much larger mosaic that is the penal community. Nevertheless, such is the chaotic, anxiety-driven politics of prisons that it does, I think, provide a template for wider understanding.

The incident

It was a Sunday afternoon in early autumn when I received the telephone call to tell me 'three of the prisoners have gone over the wall'. This news was shocking. The prisoners had broken through a fence, in fact. The fence, in a compound only used at weekends for special exercise, and with an area out of the sightline of security staff, had been breached through use of a metal structure that should have been inaccessible to prisoners.

This was a terrible and alarming affair, three serious offenders had escaped and were on the loose for a day. Fortunately they were captured before they were able to commit further offences, but it was clear that the whole security framework of the establishment would have to be reviewed.

A year after this event, almost to the day, on arriving at work I found my colleagues, the uniformed prison staff, shocked and, in many cases, in tears. Over the weekend there had been a search of the prison that began on my wing. The cause of the problem was a small craft tool that had been used for many years to carve intricate shapes in eggs that were then decorated. Many prisoners had developed great skill in making these 'fabergé' eggs. The tool had been brought onto the wing from a workshop in another part of the prison, as had been the practice for some time, so that a prisoner could continue to work over the weekend. It was shown to the staff as he arrived on the wing and on this occasion the prison officer on duty quite legitimately thought to refer this to the security department. (Although *see* Chapter 11 for an illustration of how different narratives emerge from different actors.)

What happened after that became the subject of much argument but little rational examination or debate. What is agreed is that a security operation swung into motion and the prison was searched in a way and to a degree that was unknown at this particular establishment with its long history of constructive and well ordered activity. Many of the uniformed staff and most of the prisoners were taken aback by the way the search was conducted. Curtains were torn down, many items of furniture and personal belongings were taken, even, in one particular case, a plaque that had been on the wall since the prison was built was removed and taken away. The prisoners were kept locked up for several days. The psychological and psychotherapeutic staff, highly involved in the operation of the institution, were not consulted or informed although this would have been normal practice at the establishment.

This kind of search was very unusual at the prison, where all the men had requested to come and partake in therapy to help them reduce their offending behaviour. General behaviour was good and there was a very low level of illicit drug use and of violence and bullying. In this context the reaction seemed extreme and marked a serious breach between the operational and therapeutic management.

Between these two major events, the escape and the search, this internationally renowned therapeutic prison had struggled to maintain direction. The whole period, a year, coincided with the retirement of a long established and highly respected operational governor and the promotion to another establishment of the consultant psychiatrist responsible for the therapeutic activities. In fact, the escape took place on the last weekend of the retiring governor while the search occurred a year later on the weekend that a new governor arrived. An extraordinary set of coincidences.

Sigmund Freud, who followed his father in having a lifelong addiction to cigars, is often quoted as saying, 'Sometimes a cigar is just a cigar,' suggesting that sometimes things are just what they seem, with no hidden meaning. Actually, it is difficult to establish the veracity of this quote. If Freud did say it, he said it in response to a question during a lecture tour in the United States. And if he did say it he was clearly in denial of the significance of his addiction, which was a cause of the cancer of the mouth and throat which was eventually to kill him (Elkin, 2005). So my suggestion is that the events outlined above were not isolated from each other but that one led inexorably to the other. During this period of transition the prison became more tense and felt less emotionally safe.

However, it is important to register that something was seriously disturbed at the prison during this time and, on reflection, it is rare for such humane establishments to survive the trauma of major security scares or, if they do survive, to do so without being stifled or changed out of recognition (see Chapter 1). It is even more unusual for total institutions, like prisons, to be able to have reflection and debate outside the volumes of an official enquiry, as, for example, in the case of Blantyre House (Select Committee, Blantyre House, 2001). Indeed it has been difficult to have that open debate and operational managers have understandably been keen to establish stability and control. But the debate is beginning (see Chapter 11) and this chapter is a contribution which attempts to broaden our understanding of organisational dynamics within such highly complex and dangerous total institutions.

Ramifications

It is easy to imagine any ordinary citizen or manager reading this chapter with a considerable degree of horror. The primary purpose of prison is, after all, to deprive of liberty those who offend against the rules and regulations of a given social group. This is done in order to protect the safety of the majority who remain outside. To fail in that purpose is serious indeed, to allow serious capital offenders to escape is well beyond the bounds of what is tolerable. It was expected, therefore, that there would be an investigation into these events and that changes needed to follow. Although it was never said directly, nor complaints laid, the structural changes that followed produced the impression that it was the therapeutic practitioners who were mainly being held responsible for the escape and who thus had to be brought into line. This puzzled me at first. After all, I was not responsible for the maintenance and supervision of the prison perimeter, which had been chronically neglected over years. In fact, I had never been into or seen the fenced compound from which the escape was made. That was not my job as a clinician and there were units at local, district and national level specifically charged with these responsibilities. Furthermore, I was acutely aware of the dangers intrinsic to working with a group of prisoners consisting of murderers, sex offenders and robbers, that is, with people whose lack of capacity to be contained within boundaries or observe conventional rules had been demonstrated over a lifetime. My reliance on a safe environment in order to work was absolute and I knew that I had a contribution to make to that but that I was dependent upon my operational colleagues for physical security and for protection should an emergency arise. Finally, the wider institution played a part in the situation. The prison service operates supra-establishment security procedures to ensure that security is maintained at the correct level and this had failed to see or act upon the weakness in the fence around the playing field.

However, I came to appreciate that as a clinical manager and therapist I was as responsible as anyone and that we were all in it together. There had been a breach of the physical security but there had also been a breach of the dynamic security. Dynamic security is the atmosphere of engagement and goodwill that enables two apparently opposing sides, gaolers and prisoners, to get on together and focus on a common task – in this case, the safety and security of the establishment and the pursuit of therapeutic activity. If this is effective and there is a basis of trust between staff and prisoners, this can have quite dramatic effects, such as:

- reduction of assaults between prisoners and on staff;
- improved intelligence-gathering;
- reduction in acts of indiscipline;
- reduction in escapes;
- improved use of education and other regime opportunities (Morris, 2001).

It is important to stress that the majority of prisons run with the consent of prisoners and could not operate without this consent. The greater the level of trust and respect that can be engendered, the more effective and efficient the regime can be. However, dynamic security is always transient and unstable when working with high-risk offenders. One or several men can compromise or bully more vulnerable individuals and this may take time to discern and reverse if the flow of communication is curtailed.

If a prison officer fails to notice a hole in the perimeter wall then this is an error. If a psychotherapist misses a therapeutic hole in the wall that is equally as error, particularly if he has been drawn into believing that the patients (in this case a group of prisoners) are trustworthy. In fact, none of us is trustworthy in this way, whether we are stretched out as a therapy patient in analysis in Hampstead, London or in a therapeutic group in a prison. We are all full of conflicting feelings, impulses and desires, and the job of the psychotherapist is to be aware of the weakness and vulnerability that accompanies this and so to trust and to not trust at the same time. The object must always be to pursue sceptical enquiry in full awareness of the maelstrom of conflicted feelings and impulses that are continually coming from the prisoner/patient, testing out meaning, boundaries and how he is being received. To be distracted from this focus is to be lulled into a false sense of security.

Prisons in context

Prisons are complex organisations. Invariably, individual prisons are part of a wider network of prisons, usually with a leadership cadre of governors or directors operating from a centralised office. This network of organisations will be located within a social, financial and political structure which is beset by its own peculiar set of pressures and anxieties. Politicians make reasonable enough demands upon the prison service but give insufficient resources to meet these demands. Such demands characteristically include a requirement to keep costs to a minimum, to prevent escapes and to stop convicts reoffending when they are released from prison. These expectations are often sternly enforced and staff may be moved, demoted or fired if they are considered to have failed (Travis, 2005). Thus the leadership cadre is especially sensitive to fluctuations and changes of external pressure since these may lead to loss of bonus at minimum and quite possibly dismissal. Of course, in a sense this is quite reasonable but it produces a paradox. To produce a humane environment and therapeutic benefit it is necessary to be able to allow some risk within the security of the perimeter wall. But it is commonly believed that in order to increase security the regime must be more rigorous and the security more stringent and that usually means more oppressive. This in turn attacks the contract between staff and prisoner, increasing levels of discontent and bad behaviour.

The other feature of prison-related work is that staff, especially at ground level, are dealing with the most dangerous, disturbed, disabled and socially disadvantaged people in their communities.

This is a potent combination. At one end of a continuum are politicians driven by public anxiety, fear and sometimes prejudice. Underneath the weight of this are a succession of managers and junior managers down to the coalface grades who have to respond to the pressure of these concerns while being in close contact with highly disturbed and often highly charged personalities, the prisoners. To make matters even more difficult there is an expectation that these most pressurised and least well paid and supported staff deal with their charges in a proper and decent manner. An example of this is the stance of the English Prison Service on decency:

> The Prison Service is dedicated to treating prisoners with decency in a caring and secure environment. This is a very important area of our work and requires our staff develop positive relationships with prisoners. We believe that by treating people with decency, they will be more likely to go on to live useful and law-abiding lives that will benefit them as individuals and society as a whole.
>
> We are committed to ensuring that staff, prisoners and all those visiting prisons or having dealings with the Prison Service are treated fairly and lawfully irrespective of their race, colour, religion, sex or sexual orientation.
>
> (Prison Service Website)

Laudable though this is, it presents no easy task. Not only are convicts reviled loud and long, particularly in the popular press, but prisons are places where high levels of violence and sometimes quite horrific incidents occur. In March 2000, Zahid Mubarek, a 19-year-old first offender, was battered to death in his cell within days of his forthcoming release (Ahmed, 2005). He was killed by a man with known racist views and the prison service was later found to have been negligent. In January 2004, at Lewis Prison in Arizona two prison officers were taken hostage by a couple of convicted murderers. The prisoners had nothing to lose – neither had any hope of being released from prison – and they subjected the prison officers to 15 days of terror and sexual abuse. The remarkable thing was that this siege, one of the longest in US history, ended without loss of life (Bommersbach, 2004). This was because of the determined period of extended negotiation that the Director of Corrections, Dora Schriro, insisted upon rather than the usual approach of storming the tower where prisoners and hostages were holed up. Of course, it is an all too frequent occurrence for correctional staff to lose their lives in the course of their duties in the United States. Over 14 000 correctional officers have lost their lives since 1794 and many states maintain a website in memory of their fallen employees (see, for example, Florida Department of Corrections; American Federation of State, County and Municipal Employees; New York Correction History Society). In the mind of every prison or correctional officer will be the fear that they may one day fail to stop some horror occurring or that they will be caught up in an act of catastrophic violence themselves. How difficult it must be to contain the quite normal feelings of anger, fear, disdain and hatred in relation to their charges.

A further difficulty with campaigns and exhortations to staff, such as that on decency above, is that they can drive powerful forces underground. There is a legitimate desire to reduce and eliminate unacceptable behaviours in prison staff, such as the expression of racist views or ill treatment of prisoners. However, there is the problem of what happens to the feelings which give rise to these behaviours if they are simply prohibited, since they are intrinsic to people and an expression of a powerful social norm arising from fears and insecurities. While the acting out of feelings of hatred or racial tension towards prisoners should not be allowed, unless there is some facility for powerful feelings of hate or even love to find expression, to be admitted and spoken about, then they will emerge in some other form. This may be in the form of violence towards prisoners (Dodd, 2003) or in the forming of compromising relationships between staff and prisoners.

The impact of stress in populations

We have some knowledge of what occurs to populations when they are under levels of stress, and Figure 4.1, which was actually drawn following the war in Kosovo, illustrates this. Mostly people perform best when under a reasonable degree of pressure and this is represented in the normal distribution graph, first in the series below. As tension, pressure and deprivation increase, the population tends to be driven from the centre towards the two extremes, and in a state of war this is exacerbated and the extremes become the norm with a particular increase in the tendency towards fight or flight. Characteristic of these extremes and the states of mind that they represent is an alteration in the way of thinking. A depressive thinking state is usually slowed up with a tendency to perseverate around a single matter without achieving resolution. On the other hand, fight/flight tends to produce quick-fire thinking and action. This may mean a reliance on instinct or learned behaviour or, at its best in disciplined services, acting according to order or practice.

It could be argued that, in prison populations, both staff and prisoners usually exist in the second and the third of these states of mind. Erwin James (*see* Chapter 3) clearly tells of the need to survive as being paramount, while Kimmett Edgar (*see* Chapter 6) describes in great detail the importance that violence occupies in the life and social structure of prisons.

Every now and again a prison and a prison service will shift from the second state to the third state, equivalent to a state of war, when there is a fight, a murder or rape, or if there is an escape. All levels of the institution are traumatised by such incidents. If you are present during one of these events the effect is tangible. There may be frenzied panic around a violent event or the uncanny stillness in the aftermath of an escape when prisoners may be locked up for days on end.

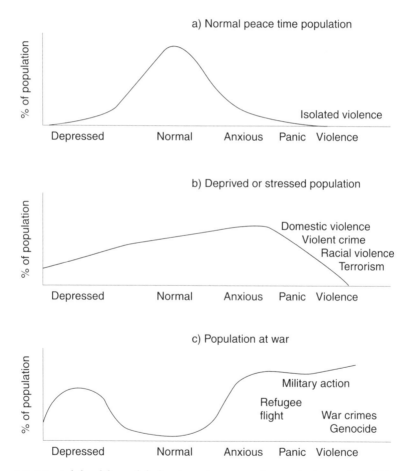

Figure 4.1 Mental health and behaviour in stressed populations: the shift to fear, violence and despair (Williams, 1999).

These dynamics will be replicated at every level. The director or governor will be in fear of losing his job and the politicians will be desperately seeking to shift the blame in order to avoid disgrace and the end of a career. The events surrounding the escape of three prisoners from the high-security prison, Parkhurst, in the United Kingdom, in 1995, are an example of this. The governor of the prison was suspended, the Director of the Prison Service eventually resigned and the minister in charge, Michael Howard, suffered public humiliation which cast a shadow over the remainder of his career as Home Secretary (Travis, 2005).

How are organisations organised?

There are many schools of management style and it can often seem that ideas come into fashion as rapidly as they disappear. The adoption of a new approach can reinvigorate an organisation that has lost direction or energy, but sometimes it can be an irritating interruption to an already productive body arising from the misguided ambition of newly arrived individuals or a directive from above. Predominant in the criminal justice system and public services generally has been the development of managerialism or the New Public Management.

Raine and Willson describe it well:

> ... a three-pronged strategy was employed; cash limits and emphasis on efficiency to engender a more financially aware and prudent approach; greater standard-isation in policies and practices to curb the autonomy of the professionals and reduce their idiosyncrasies; and reorganisation of the agencies into stronger hierarchies, supported by target setting and performance monitoring to effect greater control and to sharpen accountability.
>
> (Raine and Willson, 1997)

Managerialism has had significant beneficial effects but there are problems (Genders and Player, 1995, p. 205). The practice of expecting more for less money tends to lead to standardisation and the undermining of exceptional practice as services revert to a norm. The enforcement of target-setting and performance management can produce a culture of caution and blame which can inhibit organisational learning (Vince and Saleem, 2004). Jackson states:

> So if you are living in that hyper-defensive way it is almost like a marriage that has gone wrong. Love keeps no records, but when holy wedlock turns to unholy deadlock records are kept, and so we know that every single thing we say we have to be prepared to defend in court. And if there is supposed to be a piece of paper and there isn't a piece of paper then there are problems. If the piece of paper isn't completed correctly there are problems. Now, if we have to go down to chapter and verse, line and phrase and where the punctuation mark is, that's all very fine, but it will get you a different kind of person as a case manager. The person who rises in a situation like that will be the person who can best survive, and the person who best survives will be the person who really deals with the paperwork very well and is foolproof. There's no question that it gets to be CYA because your ass is right out there with every decision.
>
> (Jackson, 2002, p. 91)

However, regardless of management trends, organisations develop sophisti-cated but dysfunctional ways of dealing with the work they are required to do and with other, sometimes less explicit, expectations. Prison services have always attempted to be meticulous in their approach to work so that at the very least somebody makes sure that the gate is locked at the end of the day! However, meticulousness may easily segue into obsessional bureaucracy. This tendency has been fuelled by computerisation, the development of target-led management systems and offender management systems. Vast amounts of time are devoted to feeding information into computers for others to monitor and respond to.

> This system is the tail wagging the dog as it stands now. One time late last fall on one of those foggy days I looked out of the window of my office late in the afternoon. It was getting very foggy and it was getting fairly dark at that point, and I went into the Co-ordinator of Corrections Operations Office and I said, 'Norm, don't you think it's about time you should be giving some thought to locking the jail down?' He was busy working at his computer and he looked out of the window and said, 'Oh my God.' I've had visions that one day I'll be sitting in my office watching inmates jumping the fences and I'll be the only one noticing it because everyone else is dutifully working away at their computer, putting information into it . . .
>
> (Jackson, 2002, p. 93)

Such is the concern to be seen to be performing at least safely or to the minimum required level, each new challenge or crisis may be responded to by introducing a new 'system' and each new manager who wishes to impose his or her mark or have an effect may do so by 'creating' a new system. However, these often do not have the effect that is intended, as Owers describes in this volume (*see* Chapter 15). For example, introducing a new system for monitoring a prisoner who is liable to harm himself may cause staff to become preoccupied with completing the forms at the right time and in the right fashion rather than paying proper attention to the vulnerable individual. The temptation for prisons in a time of crisis is always to reduce activity as far as possible, keep prisoners locked up and monitor and record everything that they and staff do. This may be just the wrong thing to do with vulnerable self-harming prisoners. The Tavistock Institute of Human Relations, London, took a specialised interest in the anxieties arising for nurses in hospitals and the structures that typically developed to counter these anxieties.

- *Splitting up the nurse–patient relationship.* The working day of the nurse was broken down into a list of tasks that minimised her contact with individual patients. The massive increase in bureaucracy and red tape in prisons mimics this.
- *Depersonalisation, categorisation and denial of the significance of the individual.* Nurses would talk about patients not by name but by bed number or illness. In prisons, numbers or last names are often used.
- *Detachment and denial of feelings.* Seen as an important or even essential quality to avoid 'conditioning'. This is often an issue in prisons where friendliness with prisoners can be understood as a security risk. In fact, there are whole training courses on the subject of conditioning and in most impersonal, understaffed prisons they are highly relevant. However, the very best way to avoid the risks of conditioning is to establish a staff team

with a culture of openness and mutual support where the nuances of each relationship are available for discussion.

- *The attempt to eliminate decision-making by ritualising task performance.* In prisons, the preparation of audit procedures and checklists or the manualisation of treatment programmes are attempts to reduce the stress of decision-making; as are:
- *Reducing the weight of responsibility by checks and counter-checks.*

These devices appear to be attempts to solve the problem of emotional contamination arising from working with sick people and yet the rate of sickness among nurses and other disruptions suggested that the problem was only partially solved at best (Menzies, 1960). The point is that these are defensive structures and usually have their direct parallel in prisons. Such procedures may sometimes make matters worse, with staff feeling infantilised and humiliated by the lack of discretion or real responsibility they are allowed in their jobs. Patients or prisoners suffer as they receive a lower quality of interaction. Furthermore, the introduction of targets intended either to improve performance or increase production may have a particularly demoralising and damaging effect. Staff can feel that it is meeting the target rather than genuinely good performance that is the object of the exercise. More worrying is that even good and normally honest managers can feel a pressure to manipulate the figures and in that way the process can be corrupting.

A different way of thinking about these things

While it is crucial to act in 'command mode' sometimes, for example when an attack is in progress or an escape is about to take place, if that mode of thinking and behaving becomes paramount it tends to continue. Generals do not usually hand over power willingly. The effect of over-control can be stultifying and contribute to the development of a culture that fosters higher levels of violence, drug taking, bullying and self-harm. Furthermore, experience clearly shows that, although prisons and correctional facilities try very hard to improve matters through the introduction of protocols and procedures, accreditations and audits, these seem to have relatively little impact. Mission statements and other such devices may instead feed into a prevailing mood of cynicism and demoralisation on the shop floor that is only lifted by the occasional bout of frenetic activity when a fight occurs or a security alert evokes a response. One has to consider what else is at work, such as the unconscious processes within an organisation.

Bacons, screws, fraggles, nonces and scum

'Is he one of us?' Margaret Thatcher's famous test of suitability sets out rather well the basic premise of the psychological process of splitting. Mrs Thatcher was not alone in wanting to feel comfortable with her colleagues, of course, but the phrase illustrates how comfort, or relief from anxiety, can be gained by establishing difference or similarity. 'One of us' indicates that the template was already established in her mind, and her other well known comment,

'I usually make up my mind about a man (*sic*) in ten seconds, and I very rarely change it,' suggests that it could be quite difficult for anyone to shake themselves free from the model she projected onto them, particularly if it were negative. In prison one sees this splitting in staff groups:

> The communication lines between management and the operational staff were not good because the senior officers had a vested interest to keep the rest of us angry at the administration and they did that very effectively. So far as the rest of us were concerned, the senior officers were the real bosses. The management, the warden, the assistant warden and all of those people were just interlopers that didn't know what the hell they were doing. That was the prevailing attitude. It was a terribly unhealthy attitude.
>
> (Interview with Dave Sinclair, Matsqui Institution, 16 August 1993)
>
> (Jackson, 2002, p. 80)

This account from a Canadian prison is fairly typical of prisons generally.

Splitting is also demonstrated in the designations that are the linguistic currency of prison life. Bacons, Screws, Fraggles, Nonces and Scum are just some of the terms used to describe people in prison. They are not all applied to prisoners and not all by prisoners.

These terms have been stripped of humanity and when applied to individuals serve to degrade them to the level of despicable objects. With this dehumanisation may come the opportunity for a perpetrator to find violent relief from a painful sense of guilt. This occurs through a part of his own internal experience, which may, for example, be the part that is attracted to pretty little girls, being projected on to his victim who becomes (in his mind) not just deserving of attack but in need of annihilation. The greater the violence inflicted the greater the strength of the guilt which accuses, and so the cycle continues (Wilson, 1986). Sex offenders are frequently the target of such processes in prisons and in society generally.

In simple terms, prisoners are terrified of the parts of themselves that threaten the equilibrium of their ego structure. This might be to do with homosexuality (Jones, 2004), rapacious feelings about children or women, or madness. These are terms in widespread use, bacon and nonce referring to sex offenders, fraggle implying a dangerously weak mental structure, screws being prison officers and scum the term used by some staff about prisoners. Prisons can be such emotionally volatile places that these dynamics are dangerously close to the surface but they also operate at an unconscious level. Hinshelwood (2005) describes this situation.

> A split off piece of experience comes adrift from one person and is projected as if it were a package, a discrete quantum of experience . . .
>
> . . . something of the person is swept away into the group or institutional activity. Its unconscious character leads to the familiar experience of institutions as impersonal, faceless and monolithic.

Staff become involved in these feelings and more sensitive staff may experience severe emotional conflict as they attempt to resolve the demands of their conscience and their unconscious drives. At a conscious level there is the conflict induced by the clash of more scurrilous public opinion and the decency agenda previously mentioned. Less sensitive or more disturbed staff may resolve their conflict by treating prisoners badly, and often toughness and rudeness are regarded as virtues in prison. Psychologists, therapists and more sensitive staff generally may be dismissed as 'care bears' and ignored or bullied. This kind of splitting occurs at all levels of prisons' organisation.

You can't get it right all of the time

The Blantyre House Raid (Blantyre House, 2000)

In May 2000, 84 prison officers in full riot gear raided a resettlement prison in the south of England. A couple of hours previously the governor and deputy governor had been removed and a new governor installed who was then ordered to request the search. The search used considerable force and much damage was caused.

The official reason given for the search was:

> In the weeks leading up to 28 April, emerging intelligence was building up into a worrying picture of possible security breaches, concerns that prisoners may be involved in criminal activities and the emergence of inappropriate work place-ments . . . the activities the intelligence pointed to were sufficiently serious to jeopardise the protection of the public, the security of the prison and its resettlement work

> (Blantyre House Prison, 2000)

The normal expectation upon the emergence of such security information would be for the governor to be consulted, and if necessary a search would be carried out by the prison's own staff. Until this time Blantyre House had been a fine example of a resettlement prison[1] with a low rate of reconviction and excellent relations between staff and prisoners. The search found a small amount of cannabis, some pornography and a couple of mobile phones. Although these were later cited as justification for the raid, anyone who has had any contact with prisons will know that this was a very small find indeed. The damage done was considerable, financially, to the physical fabric of the prison, and to the level of trust that had been established in the prison. One prisoner said:

> They [the staff] were completely up for it, they charged into the rooms shouting, 'F***ing get out of your cell you c***!!'

> (Cohen, 2000)

Such abuse, although almost invariably denied in official reports, is common when search teams get excited and out of hand, though quite different from the usual behaviour of the same prison officers.

So what caused this event? The English Parliamentary Committee was scathing in its criticism of the prison service and the Prisons Minister was sheepish in his defence. What seems to have happened is that the Area Manager of the prison was not in sympathy with the liberal approach of the prison or its governor even though both received repeated praise from the Prisons Inspector and the Head of the Prisons Service. The security informa-tion he received came from the, perhaps ironically named, Chaucer Group, a small group of staff located in another prison. He acted upon some information, not publicly disclosed, and for several weeks planned the removal of the governor and the ensuing search.

The search and the public outcry that it provoked was a great embarrassment for the British government and prison system but it is important to consider why it happened in the way that it did. The Area Manager clearly had some anxiety about the style of the prison regime and the risk that it posed. Indeed, he extended his concern to all three of the resettlement prisons in the country. It is a common stereotype that 'care bears', strong advocates of decency and rehabilitation, are gullible and hardly competent in basic prison skills. If this were always true such people would pose a real risk. But there is a complicated equation between humane regime and security. There is considerable evidence that a decent, humane regime produces better behaviour and good security (Jones and Shuker, 2004) but if procedures are lax then eventually they will be exploited. However, for the structure to be balanced, there has to be a system that can contain the anxiety produced within the structure.

Crucially perhaps, there was a difference, amounting to a serious disagreement, about the purpose of the prison. The Area Manager saw Blantyre House as a Category C prison, for prisoners who can't be trusted in open conditions but who are unlikely to try to escape, whereas the prison governor saw it as a resettlement prison with an active programme of preparation for release leading to working in the community.

Containment

The prison service management structure is based upon a military, line management, style. There is the germ of the idea of containment in this structure in that each more senior staff member is responsible for the work of those below. However, this style is best suited to reach quick answers to questions and to resolve situations and is not conducive to the containment of anxiety other than in the very short term. There is a saying in the prison service that the primary skill for staff is to be able to say anything, concede anything, in order to get a prisoner behind his door, because then it is safe. Of course, if this really represents the level of trust and honesty that exists then the safety is likely to be short-lived.

Real containment means having a manager who can:

- hear and understand the anxieties, fears and concerns of staff even when these are not expressed and may not even be perceived;
- hold on to these feelings and think about them with the member/s of staff;
- question and resist action until the situation is clear;
- consult when doubt exists;
- feed back the concerns and fears in a form that has been modified and moderated or act in a manner that is mediated by the above procedures.

Resolution

The Incident

If we now return to the introductory paragraphs of this chapter, the incidents can be seen as a multilayered phenomenon. There had been a long period of relative stability under the leadership of a distinguished and well liked governor. He had managed to protect the culture of the institution from the effects of budget reductions, and retain a multidisciplinary approach in a service that had become a forensic psychology monoculture (McGuire, 1995; Vennard *et al.*, 1997; Downie and Jones, 2004).

The staff mainly felt their prison to be different from other prisons and, to some extent, setting an example. While the prison was sometimes referred to as the 'Jewel in the Crown' (Genders and Player, 1995, p. 202) of the English prison estate, there was not much practical evidence of appreciation. The regime was run on a shoestring, the physical structure of the buildings and perimeter wall were seriously neglected, and when the time came for massive investment in the new facilities for the treatment of those considered to be possessed of a 'Dangerous and Severe Personality Disorder' the prison was overlooked. So, within the staff group there was rather a suspicious attitude prevailing and within the prison service there were highly ambivalent feelings.

At the time leading up to the escape, along with and perhaps in reaction to this sense of paranoia ,there was an over-idealisation of prisoners in operation, into which all personnel seemed to be drawn. Through this, the idea of trust dominated, in contra-distinction to the prevailing culture of distrust elsewhere in the prison service. Thus the staff (all staff) became selectively blind in the collusive belief – a pairing in psychoanalytic terms – that they could combine with the prisoners in solving their problems.

The larger trauma

The prison service may be understood as a large organism which suffers a shock when assaulted at any point. The initial spasm may be sharp and severe, characterised by action with little time for thought. The escape of three prisoners, which occurred two years after the Blantyre House raid, represented just such a trauma. In this context, the big and unusual search a year later was both an attempt to readjust, to set matters right, and a retaliation. In both situations key players had been excluded from discussions about the process: these were the 'care bears' who, through anxiety-fuelled projections, appeared in a new and dangerous light.

Conclusion

Prisons and prison services struggle to maintain stability while attempting to resolve a mass of conflicting forces. These are just a few examples:

- political pressure for punishment versus rehabilitation;
- decency versus punishment and a desire for retaliation;

- efficiency versus chaos;
- cost cuts versus effective treatment.

The anxiety engendered within these systems is considerable and generally there is a cultural disinclination to notice this. Through the psychological process of splitting and projection, prisoners can be seen as bad: they become the holders of the badness in society and we can feel relieved that that badness is safely locked up and does not exist in us. Prisons and the prisoners manage a national anxiety (Smith, 2006). Similar splitting can occur within staff groups, between security and 'care bears', for example. In this, one side becomes invested with characteristics of harshness and the other can be seen as 'purist' or not living in the real world, so can readily be sidelined.

While there is some reality in each of these positions they are also fantasies and so the characteristics become polarised and exaggerated. These splits will occur at every level of the managerial and political structures so the task of reconciling the differences is large and difficult.

As far as prison services are concerned I advocate the following:

- There should be clarity about standards for humane prisons (Liebling, 2004; Coyle, 2003).
- There should be a policy of transparency with exceptional but clear guidelines for the requirements of security managers.
- Non-prisons professionals should have positions in prison wings. Typically these would be health or therapy staff who are able to have an independent voice. They would not usually be forensic psychologists, who do an excellent job but often have a symbiotic relationship with prison cultures. (Decaire, 2004).
- There should be an awareness that prisons and prison services will often flip into dysfunctional thinking and behaviour patterns and that special consideration needs to be given to understanding and countering these on an ongoing basis. This might include the appointment of a standing support group to operate at the highest management levels. Such a group would comprise members from psychology, forensic psychotherapy and management consultancy.

These would be difficult ideas for prison services to take on board, particularly as they could be misinterpreted as both dangerous and indulgent to staff and prisoners. However, quite apart from issues relating to moral standards, the clear evidence is that the implementation of these points could produce substantial savings in terms of staff wastage, overall costs, prisoner behaviour and reconviction. (Farringdon et al., 2001; Clarke et al., 2004)

References

Ahmed M (2005) First phase of the Mubarek inquiry Community Care 21.3.2005. www.communitycare.co.uk/Articles/2005/10/24/48645/First+phase+of+the+Mubarek +inquiry.html.

American Federation Of State, County And Municipal Employees (AFSCME). In Memorium. www.afscme.org/scripts/acu_link.pl?LastName=&Year=&State=+& Industry=Corrections&Cause=+.

Blantyre House Prison (2000) *Home Affairs Fourth Report*. HMSO. London. www. publications.parliament.uk/pa/cm199900/cmselect/cmhaff/904/90405.htm – a12.

Bommersbach J (2004) Arizona's Prison Boss. *Phoenix Magazine*. **December**. www. janabommersbach.com/pm-fea-dec04.htm.

Clarke A, Simmonds R and Wydall S (2004) *Delivering Cognitive Skills Programmes In Prison: a qualitative study*. Home Office Online Report 27/04. HMSO, London. www.homeoffice.gov.uk/rds/pdfs04/rdsolr2704.pdf.

Cohen N (2000) Pros and cons. *The Observer*. **20 August**. www.guardian.co.uk/ Columnists/Column/0,,356482,00.html.

Coyle A (2003) *Humanity in Prison: questions of definition and audit*. International Centre for Prison Studies, London.

Decaire M (2004) Ethical concerns in correctional psychology. Online paper. www. uplink.com.au/lawlibrary/Documents/Docs/Doc93.html.

Dodd V (2003) Brutality of prison officers exposed. *Guardian*. **11 December**. www. guardian.co.uk/prisons/story/0,,1104506,00.html.

Downie A and Jones D (2004) Pluralism in a Monoculture. Coming to Terms. *Forensische Psychiatrie und Psychotherapie*. Ausgabe 1, 2000. Pabst.

Elkin EJ (2005) More than a cigar. www.cigaraficionado.com/Cigar/CA_Profiles/ People_Profile/0,2540,52,00.html.

Farrington DP, Petrosino A and Welsh BC (2001) Systematic reviews and cost-benefit analyses of correctional interventions. *The Prison Journal*. **81**(3): 339–59.

Florida Department of Corrections Website. Memorial for Fallen Officers. www.dc. state.fl.us/oth/memorial.html.

Genders E and Player E (1995) *Grendon: a study of a therapeutic prison*. Oxford University Press, Oxford.

Hinshelwood RD (2005) The individual and the influence of social settings: a psycho-analytic perspective on the interaction of the individual and society. *British Journal Of Psychotherapy*. **22**(2): 155–66.

Jackson M (2002) *Justice Behind The Walls*. Douglas and McIntyre, Vancouver.

Jones D (2004) Murder as an attempt to manage self disgust. In: D Jones (ed) *Working With Dangerous People*. Radcliffe Medical Press, Oxford.

Jones D and Shuker R (2004) A humane approach to working with dangerous people. In: D Jones (ed) *Working With Dangerous People*. Radcliffe Medical Press, Oxford.

Liebling A (2004) *Prisons and their Moral Performance*. Oxford University Press, Oxford.

McGuire J (1995) *What Works: Reducing Offending*. Wiley, Chichester.

Menzies IEP (1960) A case-study in the functioning of social systems as a defence against anxiety: a report on a study of the nursing service of a general hospital. *Human Relations*. **13**(2): 95–121.

Morris M (2001) Unpublished communication.

New York Correction History Society. Webpage. www.correctionhistory.org/html/ chronicl/motchan/motchan08.html.

Prison Service Website (2004) HMSO, London. www.hmprisonservice.gov.uk/about theservice/decency/.

Raine J and Willson MJ (1997) Beyond managerialism in criminal justice. *The Howard Journal*. **36**(1): 80–95.

Select Committee on Home Affairs (2001) *Blantyre House Prison. First Special Report*. 16 January. HMSO, London. www.publications.parliament.uk/pa/cm200001/ cmselect/cmhaff/139/13903.htm.

Smith A (2006) Personal communication.

Travis A (2005) Secret Home Office papers on prison row fail to clear Howard. *Guardian*. **2 March**. www.guardian.co.uk/guardianpolitics/story/0,,1428218,00.html.

Vennard J, Sugg D and Hedderman C (1997) *The Use of Cognitive-behavioural Approaches with Offenders: Messages from the Research.* Home Office Research Study 171. HMSO, London. www.homeoffice.gov.uk/rds/pdfs/hors171.pdf.

Vince R and Saleem T (2004) The impact of caution and blame on organisational learning. *Management Learning.* **35**(2): 133–154.

Williams D (1999) Fear and violence in stressed populations. www.eoslifework.co.uk/gturmap.htm.

Wilson S (1986) The cradle of violence. reflections on the perversion of meaning. *British Journal of Psychotherapy.* **3**(2): 119–23. Published in: S Wilson The Cradle of Violence (1995) Jessica Kingsley, London.

Note

1 The aim of resettlement prisons is to resettle inmates back into the community. On arrival, all inmates are classed as Category C (closed conditions) whilst they work through a programme of personal development lasting several weeks. Only when this is completed do they become Category D and have the opportunity to work outside the prison. This may be paid work or voluntary community work.

Chapter 5

How to create madness in prison

Terry A Kupers

It's worth pausing for a moment to consider how we created as much madness as exists today in our prisons. Perhaps, after exploring how we arrived at this dreadful state of affairs, we can strive to reverse the process and foster sanity, at the same time developing humane and effective prisons.

In the era of mental asylums, when individuals suffering from serious mental illness were confined in large public psychiatric hospitals, institutional dynamics came under the spotlight. Erving Goffman, Thomas Scheff and other 'sociologists of deviance' hypothesised that institutional dynamics had a big part in driving patients to regress into impotent and bizarre, aggressive behaviours while clinicians were sidetracked into self-fulfilling biases in diagnostics (Goffman, 1962; Scheff, 1966). An example of their theory: A young man is brought to the asylum by family members who consider him 'crazy.' He protests loudly that he is not crazy and in fact it is the parents who want him locked up who are actually the crazy ones. The psychiatrist interprets his increasingly loud protests as signs of the very mental illness being ascribed to him and he is involuntarily admitted to the asylum. As he realises he is being deprived of his freedom his protests become louder and more desperate. The staff take his emotional protests as further evidence confirming the diagnosis of psychosis, he is placed on a locked ward and deprived of most familiar means of expressing himself. He does something irrational such as throwing a chair through a window in order to express his outrage over being deprived of his freedom, and the staff are even more convinced of his 'madness' and lock him in an isolation room with no clothes and no pens or writing materials. Being even more incensed and more desperate to express himself he smears faeces on the wall of the isolation room and begins to write messages with his finger in the smears on the wall. Of course, Goffman and Scheff were very concerned about the self-fulfilling prophecy aspect of the staff's diagnostic process, and they warned poignantly that incremental denial of freedom to individuals within 'total institutions,' whether they actually suffer from a bona fide mental illness or not, leads them inexorably to increasingly irrational and desperate attempts to maintain their dignity and express themselves.

Today, because of recent interconnected historical developments – including de-institutionalisation, reduced resources for public mental health services and relatively less sympathy in criminal courts for defendants with psychiatric disabilities – serious mental illness is more likely acted out in prisons than in asylums (Kupers, 1999). In fact, in the USA, there are more people suffering from serious mental illness in jails and prisons than there are in psychiatric hospitals. And the bizarre scenarios enacted in correctional settings today can make the 'back wards' of 1940s asylums look tame in comparison.

Consider as an example the scenario where the disturbed/disruptive prisoner winds up in some form of punitive segregation, typically in a supermaximum security unit where he remains isolated and idle in his cell nearly 24 hours a day. In the context of near-total isolation and idleness, psychiatric symptoms emerge, even in previously healthy prisoners. For example, a prisoner may feel overwhelmed by a strange sense of anxiety. The walls may seem to be moving in on him (it is stunning how many prisoners in isolated confinement independently report this experience). He may begin to suffer from panic attacks wherein he cannot breathe and he thinks his heart is beating so fast he is going to die. Almost all prisoners in supermaximum security units tell me that they have trouble focusing on any task, their memory is poor, they have trouble sleeping, they get very anxious, and they fear they will not be able to control their rage. The prisoner may find himself disobeying an order or inexplicably screaming at an officer, when really all he wants is for the officer to stop and interact with him a little longer than it takes for a food tray to be slid through the slot in his cell door. Many prisoners in isolated confinement report it is extremely difficult for them to contain their mounting rage, and they fear losing their temper with an officer and being given a ticket that will result in a longer term in punitive segregation.

Eventually, and often rather quickly, a prisoner's psychiatric condition deteriorates to the point where he inexplicably refuses to return his food tray, cuts himself or pastes paper over the small window in his solid metal cell door, causing security staff to trigger an emergency 'take-down' or 'cell extraction.' In many cases where I have interviewed the prisoner after the extraction, he confides that voices he was hearing at the time commanded him to retain his tray, paper his window or harm himself.

The more vehemently that correctional staff insist the disturbed prisoner return a food tray, come out of his cell or remove the paper from the cell door so they can see inside, the more passionately the disturbed prisoner shouts: 'You're going to have to come in here and get it [or me]!' The officers go off and assemble an emergency team – several large officers in total body-protective gear who, with a plastic shield, are responsible for doing cell extractions of rowdy or recalcitrant prisoners. The emergency team appears at the prisoner's cell door and the coordinator asks gruffly if the prisoner wants to return the food tray, or do they have to come in and get it? While a more rational prisoner would realise he had no chance of withstanding this kind of overwhelming force, the disturbed prisoner puts up his fists in mock boxing battle position and yells: 'Come on in, if you're tough enough!' The officers barge in all at once, each being responsible for pushing the prisoner against the wall with the shield or grabbing one of his extremities. The prisoner is bruised and hurt, but when a nurse examines the shackled prisoner and asks about injuries he responds that they hardly scratched him.

This kind of 'cell extraction,' which occurs in some supermaximum security prisons as often as 10 times per week and reminds one of the scenario that sociologists of deviance described in 1950s asylums, is not the only outbreak of madness within correctional institutions. Officers in facilities of all levels of security tend to yell at prisoners and to threaten prisoners with harsh reprisals if they do not obey orders quickly or thoroughly enough. Prisoners in whom anger has mounted because of the extremity of their situation typically respond in an angry tone, perhaps meeting swearing with swearing. Or they mutilate themselves repeatedly, or they smear faeces or throw excrement at staff. With each angry, bizarre act on the part of prisoners, correctional staff become more harsh and punitive, less interested in listening to the prisoners' expressed grievances, less concerned about prisoners' pain and suffering, and more quick to respond to the slightest provocation with over-whelming force.

The recipe

The recipe for creating madness in our prisons is easy enough to explicate. One merely needs to identify the steps that were taken to reach the current state of affairs. Here is the recipe.

- Begin by overcrowding the prisons with unprecedented numbers of drug users and petty offenders, and make sentences longer across the board.
- Dismantle many of the rehabilitation and education programmes so prison-ers are relatively idle.
- Add to the mix a large number of prisoners suffering from serious mental illness.
- Obstruct and restrict visiting, thus cutting prisoners off even more from the outside world.
- Respond to the enlarging violence and psychosis by segregating a growing proportion of prisoners in isolative settings such as supermaximum security units.
- Ignore the many traumas in the pre-incarceration histories of prisoners as well as traumas such as prison rape that take place inside the prisons.
- Discount many cases of mental disorder as 'malingering'.
- Label out-of-control prisoners 'psychopaths'.
- Deny the 'malingerers' and 'psychopaths' mental health treatment and leave them warehoused in cells within supermaximum security units.
- Watch the recidivism rate rise and proclaim the rise a reflection of a new breed of incorrigible criminals and 'superpredators'.

I will briefly discuss these successive steps to madness, starting with the massive prison crowding that began in the 1970s and continued to swell prison populations exponentially until, just after the new millennium, the prison and jail population in the USA climbed to over two million. It keeps on growing. There was convincing research at the time that prison crowding caused increased rates of violence, psychiatric breakdown, and suicide in correctional facilities (Paulus *et al.*, 1978; Thornberry and Call, 1983). One had only to tour a prison to understand how violence and madness were bred by the crowding. Consider the gymnasium that had to be converted to a dormitory with bunks for 200 prisoners. A prisoner cannot move more than a few feet away from a neighbour, and lines form at the pay telephones and the urinals. With tough men crowded into a small space and forced to wait in lines, altercations are practically inevitable. The next prisoner in line begins to harass the prisoner on the phone, saying he's been on too long, the man on the phone turns and takes a swing at the other, and there's a fight. Of course, open expressions of rage and frequent eruptions of violence tend to push individuals prone to psychiatric breakdown over the edge. Often they become preferred victims of the violence. The more violence, the more madness, and the crowding exacerbates both.

The steady rise of prison crowding since the 1980s has been driven by calls for 'tougher sentences,' especially in the context of a widely proclaimed 'War on Drugs.' More defendants are put behind bars for longer terms, and a growing number of new laws require incarceration for drug use, drug dealing, and a whole list of crimes associated with illegal drugs (Garland, 2001).

As it turns out, the theory that led to incarcerating more drug users was entirely foolhardy. Prison is not good for people with a substance abuse problem. Studies show that those who enter prison with a drug problem will leave prison with the same drug problem. And, with budget cuts, the actual amount of substance abuse treatment in prison has been declining over the past two decades. Prisoners who are not provided intensive substance abuse treatment will not transcend their drug habit while incarcerated, but as many as 60 per cent to 80 per cent of those who complete an intensive drug treatment programme in the community will be 'clean and sober' after three years (Mumola, 1997). What sense does it make to 'violate' a drug user's parole and send him or her back to prison because of a 'dirty' urine on an unscheduled test? A reasonable alternative to incarceration, a drug treatment programme in the community, would require a fraction of the expense to the state, and the diversion of people who commit low-level, drug-related crimes would vastly improve the crowding problem in the prisons. Yet, from the 1980s until the present, the sentences have grown longer, drug treatment programmes have been cut, the rate of parole violation has climbed precipitously, and the recidivism rate has been rising.

The next misstep was the dismantling of rehabilitation and education programmes inside the prisons. A turning point occurred with the publication of Robert Martinson's 1974 essay, 'What Works? Questions and Answers About Prison Reform'(Martinson, 1974). Martinson ran some numbers and announced that rehabilitation programmes have no positive effect on recidivism rates. This was the research that conservative pundits and politicians had been waiting for, and they made Martinson famous as they legislated a drastic turn from rehabilitation to harsher punishments. The article Martinson published in 1979 qualifying and recanting his rash over-generalisation never received the media attention that had been showered on his earlier castigation of rehabilitation (Martinson, 1979).

In the 1979 article Martinson confessed there had been serious flaws in his 1974 methodology. He had tried correlating the presence of any kind of rehabilitation programme in a prison with the overall recidivism rate and found no significant correlation. In 1979 he argued that a better method would have been to correlate the availability of specific programmes with the recidivism rates of prisoners whose needs were matched by those programmes, and that this more nuanced research would clearly show that rehabilitation programmes are effective to the extent they are directed at appropriately motivated and capable sub-populations of prisoners. But it was too late. The argument for longer sentences and harsher punishments had already come to dominate the public discussion about crime, and consequently very little notice was given to Martinson's recantation. With calls to 'stop coddling' prisoners, prison education programmes were slashed, weights were removed from the yards, the quality of prison food declined, prisoners were deprived of materials for arts and crafts, and so forth. Later in 1979, a dismayed Martinson took his own life (Hallinan, 2001).

With crowding and the dismantling of rehabilitation and education programmes, a wrong turn was taken in American penology, a tragic misstep that has yet to be corrected and is causing irreparable harm. Frank Wood, the former Minnesota Commissioner of Corrections, commented: 'When you take away television, when you take away weights, when you take away all forms of recreation, inmates react as normal people would. They become irritable. They become hostile. Hostility breeds violence, and violence breeds fear. And fear is the enemy of rehabilitation' (Hallinan, 2001). There was a moment in the mid-1980s, when prison violence was totally out of control, when it would have been possible for corrections departments to admit they had made a mistake and to reverse the crowding while reinstating rehabilitation and education programmes. But instead of taking the advice offered by Wood and many other experienced penologists, legislators and correctional administrators decided instead to 'lock up' the prisoners they deemed troublemakers ('the worst of the worst'), and proceeded with increasingly shrill demands for absolute control inside the prison walls. The supermaximum security unit was born. Before exploring that development, I will turn to another disastrous misstep in late twentieth century penology: the incarceration of a growing number of people suffering from serious mental illness.

The Federal Bureau of Prisons estimates that at least 283 000 prisoners have significant emotional problems and are in need of treatment (Ditton, 1999). Reasons for the expanding prevalence of mental illness in correctional settings include the shortcomings of public mental health systems, the tendency for post-Hinckley (the man who attempted to assassinate President Reagan) criminal courts to give less weight to psychiatric testimony, harsher policies toward drug offenders including those with dual diagnoses (i.e. mental illness plus substance abuse), and the growing tendency for local governments to incarcerate homeless people for a variety of minor crimes.

The fact that a growing proportion of prisoners suffer from serious mental illness has not led to proportional enrichment of the mental health treatment capacities of the prisons. There is a tendency to focus precious mental health resources on those who suffer from an obvious 'major mental illness,' such as schizophrenia, bipolar disorder and severe depression. While prisoners suffering from these conditions deserve comprehensive mental health services (which they are unlikely to receive, given current budget constraints – their treatment is often limited to cell-confinement with psychiatric medications), other disorders can cause as much suffering and disability, including anxiety, phobia, obsessive-compulsive disorder and post-traumatic stress disorder (PTSD). PTSD is especially important, since we know that prisoners, on average, have suffered from a lifetime of severe traumas, including domestic violence that they witnessed or fell victim to as children, violence and death they saw on the streets, and violence experienced as adults prior to incarceration (Kupers, 2005). Then, as convicts, they experience new traumas, including beatings, sexual assaults, and time in solitary confinement. Because of inadequacies in correctional mental health programmes, oft-traumatised prisoners receive woefully inadequate treatment for PTSD and depression. All of this compounds the problem of crowding, of course, and exacerbates the madness.

Then, added to the mix, there are attempts by corrections departments to limit and restrict visiting. This can take the form of shortened hours for visiting or requiring family members to wait in long lines to see their loved ones. It can take the form of increasingly intrusive searches, which cause humiliated family members and friends to visit less often. It can take the form of severe restrictions on mail and packages from home. Or it can take the form of punishing prisoners who violate prison rules with loss of visitation – a practice that clearly violates international human rights standards. These obstacles to visitation, combined with the fact that prisons are usually built far from the big cities where most prisoners' families reside, have the overall effect of decreasing the number and quality of prison visits. Since research clearly demonstrates that prisoners who are able to sustain quality contact with loved ones over the length of a prison term are much more likely than others to succeed at 'going straight' after they are released (Holt and Miller, 1976) these obstacles to quality contact with friends and family tend to increase the general level of madness within the prisons.

Then, in crowded facilities where rehabilitation programmes are sparse and prisoners are relatively idle, the worst traumas and abuses are reserved for prisoners suffering from mental illness. It is not difficult to figure out the reasons for this unfortunate dynamic. Consider the prison rapist's options in selecting a potential victim. He wants to choose his victim well as the wrong choice might lead to lethal retaliation. If he rapes a gang member, or even a prisoner with friends, he would be forever vulnerable to deadly retaliation. But if he selects a prisoner with significant mental illness, a loner who is not likely to have friends who might retaliate, he is more likely to get away with the rape and avoid retaliation. Thus prisoners with serious mental illness, especially if they are not provided with a relatively safe and therapeutic treatment programme, are prone to victimisation by other prisoners (Human Rights Watch, 2001). In women's prisons, rape and sexual assaults are more often perpetrated by male staff, but women who have experienced earlier traumas and those suffering from mental illness are likewise singled out for victimization (Human Rights Watch, 1996). And of course the repeated traumas they are forced to endure in prison make prisoners' mental disorders and their prognoses far more dire.

By the 1980s, when the rate of violence was clearly rising precipitously in the prisons and there were too many disruptive prisoners suffering from serious mental illness, the response on the part of the corrections system to the resulting violence and chaos was to vilify the 'worst of the worst' among prisoners, the ones presumably responsible for much of the violence, and lock them up in near-total isolation (King, 1999). The supermaximum security prison, where prisoners are almost entirely isolated and idle in their cells just about all of the time, was designed to diminish prison violence. There is ample evidence that long-term cell-confinement with almost no social interactions and no meaningful activities has very destructive psychological effects, including but not limited to worsening mental disorders and extraordinarily high rates of suicide (Grassian and Friedman, 1986; Hodgins and Cote, 1991). And newer research suggests that the turn toward supermaximum/isolated confinement for a growing proportion of prisoners is not reducing the violence inside prisons (Briggs *et al.*, 2003).

Individuals in long-term segregated prison housing tend to develop psychiatric symptoms, if not full-blown decompensation, and they universally report the build-up of uncontrollable rage. Of course, even as departments of correction rely ever more on supermaximum security and other forms of punitive 23-hours-per-day cell-confinement, only about six to ten per cent of entire prison populations are in segregation at any given time. But a much greater percentage of prisoners spend time in segregation during their prison term, and the presence of harsh segregation units within a prison or prison system has a chilling effect on the entire population.

A disproportionate number of prisoners with serious mental illness wind up in punitive segregation. For some, it is a matter of their mental illness leading to irrational acts and rule violations; for others it is a matter of losing control of their emotions and getting into altercations; and for others it is a matter of breaking down only after being consigned to segregation for a lengthy period of time. I am often asked whether prisoners with serious mental illness are selectively sent to punitive segregation, or whether the harsh conditions of isolation and idleness cause psychiatric decompensation in a vulnerable sub-population of prisoners. Of course, both mechanisms are in play. The result is that whenever I tour a supermaximum security facility in preparation for testimony in class action litigation about harsh conditions of confinement or the adequacy of mental health services, I discover a very large proportion of prisoners confined therein to be exhibiting the signs and symptoms of serious mental illness.

Of course, the presence of prisoners with serious mental illness in supermaximum and other segregation units heightens the noise level and the overall chaos. Prisoners who are not suffering from serious mental illness tell me it is extremely difficult to sleep in a unit where several prisoners with serious mental illness are up all night shouting and crying. And when a prisoner with serious mental illness flings excrement at an officer and the cell extraction team comes on the unit and sprays mace on that disturbed/ disruptive individual, the prisoners in neighbouring cells experience the effects of the mace wafting into their cells even though they have done nothing to provoke an assault by the guards. In other words, the disproportionate placement of prisoners with serious mental illness in supermaximum security units tends to exacerbate the general level of pandemonium.

Then, the same conditions that worsen psychiatric disorders make treatment problematic. Psychotropic medications are not very effective when the patient is confined to a cell, the clinician has little if any opportunity to develop a therapeutic relationship or even educate the patient about the illness and the need for medications, and there are no group therapies nor psychiatric rehabilitation programmes. Yet this is precisely the situation in many jails and prisons. In supermaximum security units the psychiatrist might even be forced to interview prisoners at their cell doors with absolutely no confidentiality.

The failure of prisoners suffering from serious mental illness to respond positively to the minimal mental health treatments available in segregation settings (typically psychiatric medications with cell-confinement) is often blamed on their 'badness' or their psychopathy. Alternatively, their exacerbated mental illness and shockingly frequent attempts at self-harm are dismissed as inauthentic or 'malingered.'

Meanwhile the frustrated staff, who cannot figure out how to improve the situation, suffer massive burn-out and become all the more insensitive to the plight of their wards (Maslach and Leiter, 1997). They find themselves losing control of their tempers and resorting to ever more harsh and punitive measures in a desperate attempt to control an impossible situation. Then, in response to the harshness and seemingly arbitrary and disrespectful actions by security staff, prisoners become more disturbed, more enraged, and capable of even more bizarre actions, such as flinging excrement at staff or repeatedly mutilating themselves. The bottom line is that we seem to have reproduced some of the worst aspects of an earlier époque's snake-pit mental asylums in the isolation units of our modern prisons.

Is this kind of madness an inevitable aspect of prison life? If that were the case, there would really be little reason to think about what kinds of changes in the way prisons are run might diminish the madness. Or does a significant proportion of the madness arise from mismanagement of the prisons? If so, the situation could be improved, i.e. better management would lead to less madness. To the extent that correctional and mental health professionals throw up their hands and proclaim that the troublesome prisoners are incorrigible, there is no improving the situation. The most that can be accomplished is isolation of the troublemakers – but that really does not solve the problem, because eventually most of them will be released from prison and, without any treatment or rehabilitation, they will pose a huge menace. The next step in this cynical, failed strategy is to change the laws to permit indeterminate civil (psychiatric) hospital commitment following completion of a determinate prison term. That strategy is being pursued in many states today, but the result is that the forensic psychiatric hospitals are becoming crowded and the madness bred of prison mismanagement is beginning to infest the mental health facilities.

A better plan would be to admit that mistakes have been made and that corrective action is needed. We need to reverse each step in the recipe I have delineated for creating madness in the prisons. And the process can be reversed. At the risk of appearing overly simplistic, I can offer a very schematic outline of that reversal here.

Crowding can be reversed by effective utilisation of diversion programmes and redesigning sentencing guidelines. Mental health courts and drug courts require treatment in the community as an alternative to incarceration. Many other forms of diversion are possible. The trend toward harsher sentences can be ameliorated in rational ways to provide the kind of community treatment and rehabilitation that is needed by many of the individuals who currently populate our prisons. Of course, to accomplish this huge goal, social policies and priorities need to be re-examined. Homelessness contributes to high incarceration rates, as does unemployment. The social safety net that has been incrementally dismantled for decades needs to be strengthened and glaring social inequities need to be addressed.

Rehabilitation and education programmes in the prisons must be reinstated and greatly expanded. It's simply not fair, and not accurate, to cut the programmes that might help prisoners 'go straight' and then blame the prisoners for their failure to do so without benefit of the needed programmes.

Individuals suffering from serious mental illness in the community must be provided with not only quality treatment in the public sector; they also need supported housing, help finding work, and so forth. If this plan were effected, far fewer of them would find their way into the jails and prisons. But there will still be prisoners suffering from serious mental illness, and they need quality mental health treatment within penal institutions.

Corrections departments must support visitation in every way that makes sense. Instead of cutting down on the hours for visits and making visitors submit to humiliating searches, they should set up free transportation for families and encourage conjugal/family visits and even home leave for prisoners who do not pose a significant security risk.

Instead of segregating problematic prisoners in supermaximum security units, a richer collaboration between security and treatment staff is needed wherein the more problematic the prisoner the more creative the staff become in effecting a management and treatment strategy tailored to help that prisoner transcend his or her problematic behaviours. Of course, implicit in this notion is the requirement that staff treat prisoners with respect at all times, and take their problems and their pains seriously (Gilligan, 2001).

A lot of attention needs to be paid to the traumas of a prisoner's life – those that occurred prior to incarceration and those that occur inside prison. Given the omnipresence of trauma in prisoners' lives, education about and treatment for PTSD needs to be readily available. The harshness of prison life needs to be ameliorated, and more intensive efforts need to be made to prevent sexual assault and other forms of violence in the prisons.

While 'malingering' does occur in prison, staff need to understand its roots in the severe deprivations prisoners experience. Before questioning whether a prisoner is really hearing bona fide voices, or is really intent on committing suicide, staff need to ask themselves what has driven the prisoner to the point of contemplating his or her own demise, or what pain is causing him or her to exaggerate symptoms. In other words, to the extent malingering is an issue, it is a symptom that requires attention.

Attention to antisocial personality disorder and psychopathy can be useful in helping shape individualised therapeutic interventions. But to the extent the diagnosis of an 'Axis II Disorder' or psychopathy leads clinicians to give up on helping a dysfunctional prisoner, that diagnosis needs to be downplayed while a more effective intervention is sought. In other words, we need to stop blaming the victim's innate 'badness' for failed interventions, and we need to try harder.

Mental health treatment services need to be expanded significantly. We must work on finding places other than jails and prisons for individuals suffering from serious mental illness, but in the meanwhile those who find their way into prisons need to be provided with adequate care. They must not be consigned to isolation in punitive segregation units, rather they require comprehensive treatment in settings that maximise their safety and their motivation to comply with treatment.

When recidivism rates rise, and when a growing number of parolees are 'violated' and returned to prison, instead of blaming the prisoners for their incorrigibility, we need to interpret the trend as a failure of our prisons to 'correct,' and we need to seek better ways to manage the prisons, and better interventions to help prisoners learn what they need to learn in order to succeed as members of the community after they are released.

Of course, what I am outlining here in very abstract terms is what has been tried, and proven effective, for example in the groundbreaking work of Hans Toch with 'disturbed/disruptive' prisoners (Toch and Adams, 2002) and at Grendon Prison in the United Kingdom (Jones, 2004; Morris 2004). The ingredients of humane prisons must include staff's constantly expressed respect for prisoners and their predicament; constant stress on communication between staff and their wards as well as among staff and among prisoners; skilled interventions by security staff as well as vocational trainers, teachers, and medical and mental health clinicians; and, very importantly, a kind of perseverance and resilience that permits staff and prisoners to rebound from the inevitable mishaps and failures along the way to ending the madness and building a truly corrective prison system.

References

Briggs CS, Sundt JL and Castellano TC (2003) The effect of supermaximum security prisons on aggregate levels of institutional violence. *Criminology.* **41**(4): 301–36.

Ditton PM (1999) *Mental Health and Treatment of Inmates and Probationers.* Bureau of Justice Statistics Special Report. US Department of Justice, Washington, DC.

Garland D (2001) *The Culture of Control: crime and social order in contemporary society.* University of Chicago Press, Chicago, IL.

Gilligan J (2001) *Preventing Violence.* Thames & Hudson, London.

Goffman E (1962) *Asylums: essays on the social situation of mental patients and other inmates.* Aldine, Chicago, IL.

Grassian S and Friedman N (1986) Effects of sensory deprivation in psychiatric seclusion and solitary confinement. *International Journal of Law and Psychiatry.* **8**: 49–65.

Hallinan J (2001) *Going Up the River: travels in a prison nation.* Random House, New York, NY.

Hodgins S and Cote G (1991) The Mental Health of Penitentiary Inmates in Isolation. *Canadian Journal of Criminology.* **33**: 175-182.

Holt N and Miller D (1976) *Explorations in Inmate-Family Relationships.* Research Report No. 46, California Department of Corrections, Sacramento, CA.

Human Rights Watch (1996) *All Too Familiar: sexual abuse of women in US state prisons*. Human Rights Watch, New York, NY.

Human Rights Watch (2001) *No Escape: male rape in US prisons*. Human Rights Watch, New York, NY.

Jones D (ed) (2004) *Working with Dangerous People*. Radcliffe Medical Press, Oxford.

King RD (1999) The rise and rise of supermax. *Punishment and society*. **1**(2): 163–86.

Kupers T (1999) *Prison Madness: the mental health crisis behind bars and what we must do about it*. Jossey-Bass/Wiley, San Francisco, CA.

Kupers T (2005) Posttraumatic Stress Disorder (PTSD) in prisoners. In: S Stojkovic (ed) *Managing Special Populations in Jails and Prisons*. Civic Research Institute, Kingston, NJ.

Martinson R (1974) What Works?: questions and answers about prison reform. *Public Interest*. **3**(5): 22–54.

Martinson R (1979) New Findings, New Views: a note of caution regarding sentencing reform. *Hofstra Law Review*. **7**(2) 243–258.

Maslach C and Leiter MP (1997) *The Truth About Burnout: how organisations cause personal stress and what to do about it*. Jossey-Bass, San Francisco, CA.

Morris M (2004) *Dangerous and Severe – Process, Programme and Person: Grendon's work*. Jessica Kingsley, London.

Mumola C (1997) *Substance Abuse and Treatment, State and Federal Prisoners, 1997*. Bureau of Justice Statistics Special Report. US Department of Justice, NCJ 172871, Washington, DC.

Paulus PB, McCain G and Cox VC (1978) Death rates, psychiatric commitments, blood pressure, and perceived crowding as a function of institutional crowding. *Environmental Psychology and Nonverbal Behaviour*. **3**: 107–17.

Scheff T (1966) *Being Mentally Ill*. Aldine, Chicago, IL.

Thornberry T and Call J (1983) Constitutional Challenges to Prison Overcrowding: the scientific evidence of harmful effects. *Hastings Law Journal*. **35**: 313–53.

Toch H and Adams K (2002) *Acting Out: maladaptive behaviour in confinement*. American Psychological Association, Washington, DC.

Chapter 6

Resolving prisoner conflicts before they escalate into violence

Kimmett Edgar

Introduction

To understand how to promote safety in the prison world, the first step is to understand the sources of violence. This chapter is based on the research, over eight years, which supported our book on prison violence (Edgar *et al.*, 2003). The prisoners' names in this chapter are all pseudonymous surnames, drawn from places in England.

This chapter:

- explores the concept of social order;
- discusses the sources and effects of conflict;
- proposes a conflict-centred strategy for reducing violence.

Social order in prisons

Richard Sparks, Tony Bottoms and Will Hay defined order as stability and predictability:

> Order: an orderly situation is any long-standing pattern of social relations (characterized by a minimum level of respect for persons) in which the expectations that participants have of one another are commonly met, though not necessarily without contestation. Order can also, in part, be defined negatively as the absence of violence, overt conflict or the imminent threat of the chaotic breakdown of social routines.
>
> (Sparks *et al.*, 1996, p. 119)

Order is built on social routines, embedded patterns of interaction that are consistent with each person's expectations of others. Order can be dynamic (changing to adapt to new situations) but it must also be sustained.

Violence is the opposite of order. It is chaotic: differences are not settled through reasoning and negotiation; the extent of harm it causes is not predictable; and the high odds of retaliation mean that violence is extremely poor at restoring sustainable patterns of social relations.

Ideas about how to engineer social order are often boiled down to two: a strict, repressive approach or a liberal regime. Coercive controls, such as lockdowns and discipline, can keep prisoners separate, but this path tends to increase frustrations and resentment. Alternatively, reinforcing social controls by creating opportunities for personal responsibility can empower some prisoners to find positive roles, but for a few prisoners such liberalism would be an invitation to prey on their peers. The liberal versus repressive dichotomy assumes that the problem of prison violence is predominantly a function of discipline, and that the solution lies in how rules are made and enforced. But personal safety depends on far more than the enforcement of rules – for example, on fairness, mutual respect and a common interest in stable relations.

Fairness is the foundation of social order in two linked dimensions. First, being fair to prisoners is the moral basis on which the governors and staff can claim that legitimate authority (Woolf, 1991). Second, in a fair social structure, basic human needs are more likely to be met, and therefore conflicts are more easily resolved.

But in prison society, the use, or threatened use, of force is omnipresent. Setting aside the question of whether prisoners view the use of force by staff as legitimate, the extent of violent behaviour among prisoners can reach levels that undermine social order. Sparks' definition seems to require that fights and assaults are relatively infrequent. How prevalent can violent incidents become before social order breaks down?

The prison victimisation survey (O'Donnell and Edgar, 1998) found that one in five adult men had been hit or kicked or assaulted in some way in the month before the survey. Although the data did not provide detail about how serious the injuries were, such a high prevalence of assaults must undermine social order to some extent. But a different perspective on assault rates should be considered. The use of force by prisoners may perform particular functions in maintaining prisoner society.

Bottoms suggested that prisoner subculture is:

> . . . a special kind of social context unusually weighted towards coercive power and that [. . .] nevertheless frequently contains elements of predictability and order.
>
> (Bottoms, 1999: 275)

McCorkle (1992) and others record as an axiom of prison life that the prisoner needs to show a willingness to defend his interests with physical force if he is to avoid being targeted by others for exploitation and assault. This suggests that, for many prisoners, *'the expectations that participants have of one another'* (a central part of Sparks' definition) must include the expectation that their counterparts will use force if they are convinced it is necessary.

The term 'violence' can distort the picture because, used in this way, it ignores the valid question whether a prisoner's use of force in particular circumstances could contribute to order. Posing violence as the opposite of order implies that any use of force by prisoners is illegitimate and destabilising. Thus, part of the puzzle is to explore how the use of force by prisoners fits into their sense of social order.

The anthropologist David Riches (1986) claimed that any use of force is contestable. When force is used, judgments about its legitimacy are based on determining whether it was necessary, and whether its use was proportionate to the need. These are important questions irrespective of the status of those who use force. Riches' work suggests that for any use of force it is possible to trace different, valid perceptions. In a similar vein, Sparks and Bottoms (1995) made the point that the use of force by officers does not secure legitimacy: rather, each use of force by the staff is a test of their legitimate authority.

Prisoners recognise the legitimacy of the use of force by other prisoners in a variety of circumstances. For example, many believe that force is required when a debtor refuses to repay. The use of force to punish cell thieves or sex offenders is also sanctioned by some members of the prisoner community.

The victimisation survey found that almost three-quarters of prisoners had traded with their peers. Because trading possessions is illicit, prisoners cannot turn to staff to mediate when an exchange goes wrong. In such disputes, the use of force is seen by many prisoners as a legitimate method of regulating the activity.

A prisoner described the circumstances in which he had been assaulted: 'I found phonecards at the telephone. There was no name on them so I took them. He found out, came to my cell. "Have you got my cards?" I said no. He found out that I did, though, and came back and hit me a number of times; eight or nine times on the same spot – just punches on my arms. I gave him back the cards. Afterwards he apologised. We shook hands, had a cigarette and no more problems. I asked for it myself. He didn't want to do it, but I lied to him.' The victim of this assault viewed the use of force as a legitimate response to his attempt at exploitation.

Some prisoners used force as a form of rebellion against the authorities. Among young offenders, there is a tendency to arrange fights in advance, out of sight of prison officers (see the ESRC study by Edgar and Martin, 2000). Such conspiracies were clearly intended to circumvent the authority of officers to maintain order. But in the eyes of many young offenders, fights settled conflicts: they believed that fighting cleared the air and, in this sense, contributed to social order.

For some prisoners, violence was so widespread in their social networks that it appeared normal. The ESRC study found that nine in ten prisoners surveyed agreed with the statement, 'Violence in prison is inevitable.' When 30 per cent of young prisoners are assaulted in a month (O'Donnell and Edgar, 1998), violence may have become so widespread that it is routine. Many young offenders felt that violence was expected of them, and they were aware of the possibility that their opponents would use force. These are the characteristics of a society in which violence is conventional.

Thus force can have the functions of regulating prisoner interactions (e.g. trading); punishing those who break the code; rebellion against the authorities; or settling differences. When any specific incident is analysed in depth, the functions of using force depend partly on perspective. Consider the following example.

The prisoners on W wing suspected that Westcott was informing on them, so they set him a test. They told him that Jedburgh had some hooch in his cell. The next morning, officers raided Jedburgh's cell and searched it thoroughly. A number of prisoners on the wing were thus convinced that they had firm evidence against Westcott. Later in the day, Broadby and Daventry cornered Westcott and beat him severely.

This story illustrates the punishment, by prisoners, of offences against the prisoner community. From the officials' perspective of the need to maintain social order, a punishment beating is a break in the order because a prisoner has been physically injured by another or others.

In the prisoner community, however, the guilty prisoner has received what he deserved, justice has been done, and their sense of order – the world in which no one can betray the prisoner world and get away with it – has been *restored*. Sending a signal to other prisoners not to pass information to officers is also a rebellion against officers' power to exert control.

Broadby and Daventry defined their actions as a last resort, a necessary step to punish those who would betray the solidarity of prisoners. The punishment beating (as they saw it) was a means of regulating inmate conduct.

Different types of prison society favour particular functions of force. For example, in Young Offender Institutions, violence is more likely to be used as a convention, as evidenced by a high level of routine assaults and threats. Older, settled prisoners in adult institutions see violence as a disruption to their routine. In women's prisons, violence primarily serves to punish those who have offended against the prisoner community. For a limited number of prisoners in each type of institution, violence is a method of resisting the imposed order.

Values and social order

The prevention of violence cannot be limited to the continuum from strict to lax enforcement of rules. Fortunately, a wider perspective is available. In her 2004 book on prisons' moral performance, Alison Liebling analysed values about social order as they apply to prisons. She followed Valerie Braithwaite in suggesting that societies maintain a dynamic relationship between two sets of values: security and harmony.

The security values comprise self-protection, the rule of law, authority, competitiveness and tough law enforcement. This package of mutually reinforcing values supports a hierarchical social structure. In theory, the security model contributes to personal security via the threat of punishment by the authorities and by sacrifices in individual liberty in the interests of self-protection.

The harmony model is based on peaceful coexistence, mutual respect and human dignity, a fair sharing of resources, including wealth redistribution and an interest in the development of the individual. The priority given to peaceful coexistence suggests that this model is prepared to sacrifice the incentives that competition can provide to achieve unity among the members of the society. Personal security is achieved through the practice of respect for each other's needs rather than through coercion and dominance.

Although it might be assumed that social order in prisons is based purely on the security model, Liebling argued that a balance is set in each prison, with some giving greater weight to harmony values than others. However, the hierarchical structure of prisons, staff holding authority over prisoners at all times, implies that they are inherently places of dominance. She wrote:

> The prison is a morally dangerous environment. It is dangerous precisely because of the need for force to be used and security to be accomplished. Because power is

corruptible, and security values inevitably involve scepticism and detachment, it is extraordinarily difficult to pursue respect and security values simultaneously.

(Liebling, 2004, p. 442)

Conflict in prison society

The causes or sources of conflict between individuals and groups cannot be separated from the totality of relationships, and the environmental conditions that promote relationships.

John Burton (1990, p. 47)

Prison life is a continuing series of close calls in which violence is narrowly avoided.

Lee Bowker (1983: 29)

The main sources of violence in prison are manifold. Reducing the factors that contribute to prison violence to a single cause – like anger, or drugs, or a high proportion of violent men in the population – is inevitably superficial and simplistic.

Much can be gained from investigating prison violence as the outcome of conflicts between prisoners. Conflict can be defined as 'competing interests which the parties pursue in uncompromising ways'.

In this sense conflict is endemic in prison. Conflict may lead to violence, or it may be resolved before it escalates.

Conflicts can be analysed in terms of six components:

- *interests* (both material goods, such as tobacco, and values, such as respect);
- *relationships* (between the parties whose interests clashed, including how well they knew each other – social distance – and any power imbalance between them);
- *catalysts* (the tactics prisoners used in reacting to conflict that made violence more likely, including threats and accusations);
- *interpretations* (how each party understood their counterparts' purposes);
- *purposes* (the immediate functions the person(s) who used force intended it to serve); and
- *social context* (the contribution of the prison as a behavioural setting).

Some of the factors that contribute to violence, as deduced from detailed analyses of violent incidents in prison, include:

- poor conflict management skills, such as the use of intimidation or threats;
- theft and other forms of exploitation;
- racial and cultural tensions and misunderstandings;
- emotions, such as frustration, anger and shame;
- transitoriness of relationships, lack of familiarity with peers;
- low self-esteem, aggravated by low approval/high criticism climate.

Institutional or structural dimensions that foster these factors (the social context of violence) include:

- danger – risks of being victimised;
- material deprivations;
- powerlessness – the deprivation of autonomy;
- distance between prisoners and staff;
- lack of legitimate conflict-resolving opportunities.

Danger

Prisoners accept that there is a pervasive risk of being involved in physical violence. Their perceptions that prisons are risky settings were supported by the actual rates of assault, revealed in the prison victimisation survey.

The high levels of crime and incivilities are interpreted by many prisoners to mean that they must physically defend their possessions and personal security. Other victimisation, including insults, racial abuse and harassment, exacerbate disputes and make violence more likely. Living in prison subjects prisoners to a pervasive risk of being intimidated, exploited or injured.

Leith was in the food queue when challenged by Selby. He assaulted Selby the following day. He explained his reasons: 'I sat in my cell and thought I might as well do him before he can get to me so I put a battery in a sock and I saw him queue up for dinner and I attacked him.'

Midgley tried to intimidate Hatton into taking the blame for something that Midgley had done. But Hatton resisted. He took Midgley's threats seriously and decided to get to him first. Hatton explained: 'I said I wasn't going to take the rap. He then started to threaten me through the pipe. He threatened to cut me up and throw hot water at me if I didn't agree. I became paranoid about it. I waited till dinner time when we were unlocked and then I hit him.'

A clear distinction can be made in prison society between an individual's sense that he is threatened by another identifiable individual (as above) and a more ambiguous risk from unknown others. Some prisoners voiced concerns about appearing vulnerable to inmates not involved in their dispute. About one in four assailants was motivated primarily by the idea that a demonstration of toughness was required to ward off danger. If a prisoner assumed that potential predators would respect shows of force, then he or she was likely to grasp violence as a means of reasserting some control over their environment.

Darwen was playing pool and winning. A number of other prisoners were watching him play. Brough challenged him to a game, and they bet on the outcome. At the end of the game, they argued about who had won. Brough reacted to Darwen's claims to the winnings by threatening him: 'I'll see you upstairs.' Darwen believed that his reputation would be damaged by Brough in that other prisoners would consider him weak.

Darwen explained his interpretation: 'I'm thinking in these jails "upstairs" means serious – bottles or stuff. I'd have got whispers saying he's going to stab you, so I needed to do something there, not later.'

In response, Darwen attacked Brough with the pool cue. Darwen explained his interpretation of Brough's intentions: 'He was trying to show me up in front of other people. I've had it before a few times. I'm only small and when it starts you've got to nip it in the bud. The next day, a lot of people said, not, you were right, but, you did what you had to do. I've been in a jail before where I thought, leave it and I didn't have a fight and I was ending up having to fight a few people who thought they could do the same.'

The purpose of demonstrations of toughness was to show the other inmates on the wing – the sea of unfamiliar faces – that one could not be victimised with impunity (a kind of general deterrence). As one offender who initiated a fight explained: 'If it wasn't for the other inmates, we wouldn't have fought. Most prison fights aren't about being angry. They're about what other inmates will think of you if you don't fight.'

There is little empirical support for the belief that projecting a tough image achieves greater personal security. The prison victimisation survey showed that those who had assaulted others were more likely to be assaulted. Prisoners who feel intimidated may believe that an aggressive response will force the other inmate to back down; the evidence suggests it is more likely to initiate a cycle of violence.

The cycle of physical violence is an example of contradictory consequences. One individual feels at risk and believes that a show of force is needed to guarantee his safety. He assaults the person he fears, and in so doing, increases the amount of violence in the prison. His attempt to protect himself makes his environment more dangerous for everyone.

Living where there is a risk of being assaulted affects how prisoners respond to conflict. When a dispute is becoming tense, prisoners must be aware of the distinct possibility that the other party will use aggressive physical force. Both parties are likely to infer hostility from their foe, leading each to feel justified in preparing a violent response.

Material deprivations

Human needs encompass values and attitudes, the right to be treated with decency. But there are also physical human needs, access to which is restricted through the unnatural material deprivations in prison. While disputes arise over objects such as phone cards, tobacco or drugs, the deeper concerns such as loyalty, respect, trust and fairness probably have greater influence in driving interactions towards violent outcomes.

A society in which material goods are hard to come by, combined with a lack of respect for property, can motivate some prisoners to better their quality of life at the expense of peers. However, there is a more important bridge between the deprivations inherent in prison and violence. Things like tobacco or food symbolise deeper personal needs. As a dispute grows, these needs become more important. After punching Hastings, whom she suspected of cell theft, Didcot explained: 'It sounds silly fighting over tobacco, but you can't let it go without losing your respect. You wouldn't fight about it on the out, but we are not on the out. We're in jail.'

Powerlessness

Prisons place the prisoner at the bottom of a rigid hierarchy of power. The actions of any prisoner are subject to the scrutiny and judgment of any member of staff. With their power over their own lives so restricted, prisoners tend to be sensitive to the balance of power between them and their peers.

Lack of control over decisions fosters a sense that one must take a violent course (it is not seen as a choice). Most prisoners did not want to become violent but could not see an option in their circumstances. The power imbalance between staff and prisoners reinforces the belief that 'might makes right', and this belief makes it much more difficult to find non-violent solutions to conflict.

One of the consequences of the loss of power is that prisoners become hypersensitive to impressions that another prisoner might attempt to treat them as an inferior. The most common situation leading to violence in the ESRC study was the power contest, disputes in which the main cause of the conflict was a battle for power, one over the other. Power contests were propelled by mutual intimidation. Power contests are driven by a narrow focus on a limited range of possible responses, a belief that force decides issues of control, and win or lose thinking.

Collecting his meal, Auckland noticed a dent in his ice lolly. He asked for a replacement. The servery worker, Sowerby, told him no. Auckland replied, 'I ain't no dickhead.' He said to another servery worker that Sowerby should do as he was told and give him a replacement. Sowerby again refused, and Auckland returned to his cell.

The following morning, Sowerby was standing in front of the servery when Auckland came for his breakfast. Sowerby glared at him and asked him why he was running off his mouth. Auckland returned the stare and laughed. Sowerby went to walk away, but then changed his mind. He came back to Auckland and began punching him. An officer intervened and was injured trying to separate the two inmates.

Auckland felt Sowerby was trying to intimidate him by giving him an inferior ice lolly, staring at him and standing in front of the servery in a threatening way. Auckland explains that he laughed at Sowerby in the morning to show him 'that his looks do not scare me at all'. Sowerby felt humiliated when Auckland turned to the other worker to overrule his judgement about the dessert. Asked what effect that had on him, he said it: 'made me feel small. He was trying to intimidate me.' They both interpreted the other's behaviour as an attempt to establish superiority:

> Auckland: He was trying to take me for a fool.
> Sowerby: He was trying to put me down, like he was higher than me.

Auckland and Sowerby's mutual suspicion had a profound impact on the conflict. Each thought that the other was hostile and trying to intimidate the other. In reaction to their reading of the other's behaviour, each resorted to increasingly aggressive stances. Both participants explained that they acted the way they did to show the other person that they could not be exploited or dominated. Each set himself an objective to demonstrate his strength to the opponent. Their strategy was to use hostility to protect themselves, presumably in the hope that the other person would back down. Each judged the behaviour of the other to be aggressive. Each tried to resolve the tension between them by putting on a tough front. The decisions each made in response to the other put them on a collision course towards violence.

Distance between prisoners and staff

Misconceptions about the nature of victimisation hamper attempts to for-mulate an effective response. As so little of what goes on is reported to them, members of staff may be misled into thinking that what they do hear about is typical, and may make generalisations on this basis. There is a real risk that any intervention could be misinformed and even counterproductive if it is based on such partial information.

Few assaults, threats or frauds are disclosed to officers (O'Donnell and Edgar, 1998). The code of hiding problems creates a need to resolve problems within the prisoner community: 'You know when you don't get paid back you can't go to the governor and say, "I loaned him five burns." You got to punch him.'

Thorpe had loaned Alderly some tobacco. On association he entered Alderly's cell and picked up a few goods in compensation. Alderly entered his cell and demanded an explanation. Thorpe punched him several times, then left.

Lack of formal methods by which prisoners can resolve conflicts

Young offenders in particular saw violence as a means of resolving their conflicts. Amongst adults, violence was used to regulate their interactions when there were reasons precluding taking difficult situations to the staff.

Sutton was complaining to an officer when Whaley came up and told Sutton to shut up. Sutton immediately challenged him to a fight. They went off to the showers, but an officer intervened and sent them to their cells. At lunch they continued to exchange threats. Whaley had a visit first thing in the afternoon. When he returned to the wing, Sutton again challenged him to a fight.

Sutton described his frustration by this point in the dispute: 'Whaley came up and was threatening me, "I'm going to kill you." Talking, talking. I was getting tired of this. We had to settle this, we had to have a fight.'

A violence-prone social environment?

The conflict-generating structures of prison cultures shape the prisoners' perceptions of what the prison world requires of them. The atmosphere of distrust and suspicion in which disputes develop colours a prisoner's assump-tions about what the other person is trying to achieve.

Prisons where there are high rates of assault and threats of violence, and authoritarian or coercive control exercised by officers, fail to meet human needs for safety, rationality and a sense of control. Prisoners in such a setting might grasp violence as a means of reasserting some control over their circumstances.

Prisons with high rates of theft and robbery, or where staff take a laissez-faire attitude to the victimisation of some prisoners by others, fail to uphold prisoners' needs for a fair distribution of goods, consistent responses to behaviour and personal security. The belief that force restores order after norms have been transgressed leads some prisoners to manage these risks by inflicting punishment on suspected thieves. Hence there are strong links between material deprivation, victimisation and norms supporting retaliation that fuel many conflicts over exploitation and drive them towards a violent conclusion.

These are cycles of prison violence, mutually reinforcing influences that powerfully increase the likelihood that the prison social structure will feature institutionalised violence; that is, the perception amongst a large majority of the members of that society that violence is normal.

These cycles are exacerbated by regime factors such as a lack of useful activity. When prisoners are deprived of adequate stimulation, they may lose a sense of role and feel that they have little control over their future. The lack of incentives that jobs otherwise provide – improved standards of living, time out of cell, opportunities to prove one's reliability – means that prisoners may feel they have little to lose if they resort to violence.

A conflict-centred approach to preventing prison violence

A life sentence prisoner told us the following story:

> I was in the chapel installing a sound system. When I turned my back someone took a microphone. I saw only one other person in the chapel. So I went straight to him and confronted him. I said, 'A microphone's gone missing. Did you nick it?' He shook his head. I said, 'Well, I need to get it back or it is on me.' I went back to work and he came to me ten minutes later and said, 'What did you say?' I repeated what I'd said, and explained I wasn't accusing him, but he was the only one I'd seen so I had to ask him. He said, 'But now you're putting it on me.' And I told him, 'I wasn't accusing you, but you were the only one I'd seen.' He went away and returned with the microphone.

The episode illustrates an important aspect of reducing violence: prisoners have an interest in a peaceful environment and managers could do far more to build on this common ground, enlisting the cooperation of prisoners in finding non-violent solutions to conflict.

It is important to question the myth that locates violence as the end to a train of events. Seeing violence as part of a process helps to show that violence is often undertaken through decisions that could have been different, could have led to non-violent outcomes.

Prison staff, however, often become aware of a dispute only when its violent outcome brings it to their attention. The ESRC study interviewed 58 prison staff about their response to a fight or assault between prisoners. Half of these officers did not know what the dispute was about. When officers did not know the background circumstances, determining who was to blame was based on guesswork. Official interventions to protect an inmate labelled a victim or to punish a suspected perpetrator risked exacerbating the original conflict and led to unjust outcomes.

As a consequence of the gap of knowledge about the situations that lead to violence, policies to reduce prison violence are often based on this very limited perspective. The violent incident is the starting point for developing preventative policies. The sources remain hidden.

Not surprisingly, then, violence reduction strategies tend to be based on:

- how staff can identify prisoners with the potential for violence;
- how staff can deploy physical force to minimise injuries; and
- punishing perpetrators as a way of deterring future assaults.

None of these strands really addresses the underlying causes of prison violence, because they ignore the reasons people turn to physical force. That gap in understanding was the reason for undertaking the ESRC study.

The conflict-centred approach is proactive and multifaceted, allowing steps to be taken early, so that violence can be prevented. Managers, in consultation with officers and prisoners, can identify possibilities for reducing the sources of conflict. The key finding of our research is that the solutions lie in exploring the sources of conflict between prisoners and identifying the conditions that generate those conflicts. A conflict-centred approach implies a pioneering change in the strategies prisons use to reduce violence.

The four ingredients of an effective approach to promoting personal safety are:

- fulfilling prisoners' basic human needs;
- a focus on ensuring personal safety;
- providing opportunities for the exercise of personal autonomy; and
- building in mechanisms for prisoners to resolve their conflicts.

To build a sustainable social order it is necessary to consult prisoners, to determine which basic needs the prison is not meeting. Although the deprivation of self-determination, the denial of basic needs and the high crime rates are obvious problems, there are other sources of conflict. Prison managers who are determined to improve the service to prisoners are good at bringing conflicts to light and working with prisoners to try to find solutions. They need to be resourceful in trying to learn from prisoners what their main concerns are. Prisons should also consider using surveys to establish the concerns that are most important to prisoners. The prison that most successfully fulfils the basic needs of the people it holds will be seen as a place of legitimacy and safety.

Opportunities to exercise personal autonomy carry risks, but the clear benefit is that prisoners can begin to assume responsibility for contributing to a safe environment.

There is wide-ranging evidence that providing prisoners with appropriate means to resolve their disputes can reduce tensions and thereby prevent violence. One promising development is staff–inmate dialogue and prisoner representative meetings. These not only increase contact between staff and prisoners, providing both groups with, at times, mutual goals, but also reduce the level of tension by providing an appropriate channel for dealing with grievances.

The Prison Reform Trust's study of prisoner councils suggested that councils perform a vital function of bringing conflicts to light so that they can be worked through. A governor interviewed in that study felt strongly that starting the council had resulted in a decrease in assaults. A prisoner contrasted the atmosphere in prisons with or without a council:

> You get anger in other prisons. You walk past another con and you feel the anger welling up. Soon you feel that with every other prisoner. You feel the tension all of the time. Here, you bring it up in the wing meeting and settle it.
>
> (Solomon and Edgar, 2004, p. 25)

A key step is for the prison to turn from working in opposition to the prisoners, and begin to develop ways of working with them. Prisoners, staff and managers have a common interest in keeping prisons as safe as possible. The prison authorities should think about how to encourage this common interest, sharing with prisoners the problems, conflict and violence, and jointly developing solutions.

When the prison management team have a good idea of how they can better meet the primary concerns of the prisoner community, governors can then focus on techniques for handling conflict. This could mean training both prison staff and prisoners in mediation and other conflict-resolution skills.

Many of these principles are already in the Violence Reduction Strategy, published by the Prison Service (HMPS, 2004). However, the emphasis on identifying causes of conflict and resolving differences before they escalate into violence calls for a shift in traditional prison staff culture. It is crucial that prisons recognise the risks of slipping back into outdated methods which emphasised control and restraint and the role of officers in identifying potentially violent individuals.

What role can officers play?

Only two of the 58 officers interviewed in the ESRC study said they could have done something to prevent the violent incident; and nine in ten agreed with the statement: 'Violence is inevitable in prison'.

Prison officers interviewed felt that they had little power to influence the course of inter-prisoner disputes or to prevent violent outcomes. In training staff in the skills they need, the focus should be on:

- developing methods of handling of inmates' disputes by focusing on the interests, values and needs at stake;
- identifying aggressive tactics and confronting behaviour such as insults, threats, accusations or hostile gestures;
- improving communication between the parties;
- searching for win–win outcomes;
- striving to create a culture that favours negotiation and the fulfilment of basic human needs over coercive controls.

Effective policing of victimisation is also essential. One way to reduce assaults is to pay greater attention to preventing exploitation of prisoners by prisoners.

The strategy must also be able to empower officers to ensure safety from victimisation. Much of the victimisation that occurs – including threats of violence, thefts and assault – is criminal. Typically, a dispute between prisoners escalates from incivilities, like insults and mutual threats, to pushing and shoving, and then to an all-out fight.

Peacekeeping by staff includes:

- methods of preventing or minimising violence through . . .;
- the sensitive handling of inmates' disputes by officers by . . .;
- focusing on the interests, values and needs at stake;
- identifying the tactics each party has used and intervening to stop prisoners using tactics such as insults, threats, accusations, hostile gestures and challenges;
- improving communication between the parties;
- searching for options for win–win outcomes;

all of which must occur within a social context that favours negotiation and the fulfilment of basic human needs over coercive controls.

The enforcement of rules is central to the officer's job. Situational control is needed to ensure the personal safety of prisoners. The fact that the risk of deception, thieving and robbery should be routine in prisoners' lives highlights the serious problem faced by prison managers of maintaining safe custody. One way to reduce assaults is to pay greater attention to preventing the victimisation of prisoners.

Prisons can resolve conflicts and thereby reduce violence, but to do so, their role must shift:

- from the reactive (using force when fights break out) to the preventive; and
- from enforcing the rules to a broader more engaged sense of peacekeeping as conflict resolution.

In addition, the peacekeeping roles have training implications. Officers need specialised training:

- to recognise potentially volatile situations as they arise between prisoners;
- to know the circumstances in which it would be beneficial to intervene;
- to deal with conflict so that their interventions are not counterproductive.

Arguably the most important part of the officers' role is how they can intervene appropriately to facilitate the resolution of conflicts between prisoners.

Restorative justice also informs how prisons can change their approach to address the sources of conflict. The strategy should apply restorative principles, as follows.

First, it should be inclusive. Picking up on the sources of conflict in deprivations, representative groups of prisoners should regularly be consulted to gain an understanding of the most pressing deprivations and to decide, collectively, how some of these could be addressed.

Second, it should focus on harm rather than rule-breaking. The whole prison should focus on preventing victimisation, and respond to harmful behaviour in a way that rejects the harmful acts while seeking the reintegration of the perpetrator. On this note, the Prison Service in England and Wales is currently applying the following definition

Violence is defined as:

> any incident in which a person is abused, threatened, or assaulted. This includes an explicit or implicit challenge to their safety, well-being or health. The resulting harm may be physical, emotional or psychological.

Third, in the aftermath of violence, prisons should promote a non-punitive, problem-solving response. The routine, formal response should be a conference, facilitated by external, trained mediators, and including each party's supporters. The conference will try to establish the sources and course of the conflict that led to the violence, as a means of understanding how the problem escalated.

The current HMPS Violence Reduction Strategy, strongly influenced by proactive, problem-solving thinking, is based on this principle:

> By constructively and consistently taking action to prevent violence and promote fairness and decency, prisons can offer a structured environment in which to influence future behaviour, encourage positive communication and develop social skills that assist offenders with rehabilitation.

References

Bottoms AE (1999) Crime and justice. *Prisons*. **26**: 205-81.

Bowker, L (1983) An Essay on Prison Violence. *The Prison Journal*. **LXIII**(1): 24–31.

Burton J (1990) *Conflict Resolution and Provention*. St Martin's Press, New York.

Edgar K and Martin C (2000) *Conflicts and Violence in Prison: research findings from the ESRC Violence Research Programme*. http://www1.rhbnc.ac.uk/sociopolitical-science/vrp/Findings/rfedgar.PDF.

Edgar K, O'Donnell I and Martin C (2003) *Prison Violence: the dynamics of conflict, fear and power*. Willan Publishing, Devon.

HM Prison Service (2004) *Violence Reduction Strategy*. http://pso.hmprisonservice.gov.uk/PSO_2750_violence_reduction.doc.

Liebling A (2004) *Prisons and Their Moral Performance*. Clarendon, Oxford.

McCorkle R (1992) Personal precautions to violence in prison. *Criminal Justice and Behaviour*. **19**: 160–73.

O'Donnell I and Edgar K (1998) *Bullying in Prison*. Centre for Criminological Research Occasional Paper Number 18. Centre for Criminological Research, Oxford.

Riches D (ed) (1986) *The Anthropology of Violence*. Basil Blackwell, Oxford.

Solomon E and Edgar K (2004) *Having Their Say: the work of prisoner councils*. Prison Reform Trust, London.

Sparks R and Bottoms AE (1995) Legitimacy and Order in Prisons. *British Journal of Sociology*. **46**: 45–62.

Sparks R, Bottoms AE and Hay W (1996) *Prisons and the Problem of Order*. Clarendon, Oxford.

Woolf H (1991) *Prison Disturbances 1990: Report of an Inquiry by Rt Hon. Lord Woolf and His Honour Judge Stephen Tumim*. Cm 1456. HMSO, London.

Chapter 7

Can there be 'best practices' in supermax?

Lorna A Rhodes

In 1997 Human Rights Watch published a report entitled *Cold Storage: Super-Maximum Security Confinement in Indiana*. Based on research conducted in the wake of a class action lawsuit against the Indiana Department of Corrections, *Cold Storage* documents conditions of confinement in two Indiana facilities, including their policies and security measures, the reported behaviour of staff, and excerpts from prisoner interviews. Human Rights Watch concludes that:

> By choosing to subject hundreds of prisoners to prolonged periods in extremely harsh and potentially harmful conditions that cannot be justified as reasonably necessary to ensure security or to serve the legitimate goals of punishment, the Indiana DOC has violated the prohibition on cruel, inhuman or degrading treatment contained in the International covenant on Political and Civil Rights and the United Nations Standard Minimal Rules for the Treatment of Prisons.
>
> (Human Rights Watch, 1997, p. 11)

While highly critical, *Cold Storage* also expresses approval of a number of positive changes made by the Indiana DOC, and offers specific recommendations designed to lessen the harm of this form of confinement. Unlike the general statement above, these recommendations suggest specific policies of operation such as, for example: 'Provide frequent monitoring by qualified mental health professionals . . . to identify [inmates] who need mental health services' (*ibid.*, p. 14).

Three things have happened in the almost ten years since *Cold Storage* was published. First, an unknown number of additional supermax prisons have been built in the United States and elsewhere.[1] Some of these new facilities are, if anything, even more restrictive than the Indiana prisons described in the report. Second, more information is available about supermax confinement, much of it describing – with similar recommendations and no better resolution – the same issues raised by Human Rights Watch in 1997. And finally, the contradiction expressed in *Cold Storage* has only become more apparent. On the one hand, supermax prisons impose cruel and unusual punishment. On the other hand, it is possible to recommend simple measures that can ameliorate conditions and produce a somewhat less harsh regime without changing the basic structure of this form of confinement.

In this chapter I bring together the two sides of this contradiction. I first briefly describe supermax confinement as it is generally practised in the United States.[2] I then turn to why this form of incarceration is 'cruel and unusual' and discuss the wider context in which these facilities have become a routine part of prison construction and management despite criticism from Human Rights Watch and numerous other observers. Unfortunately, it isn't enough to stop there and argue for the elimination of these prisons. They are not likely to be emptied out any time soon. Further, as the excerpt from *Cold Storage* indicates, the development and continuing use of supermax is driven to some extent by 'reasonable goals of security' and the 'goal of punishment' as these are understood by prison administrations. While a larger rethinking of the prison complex as a whole is sorely needed, these more immediate goals drive existing prison management.[3] I describe briefly, then, some modest and relatively simple – though not easily implemented – changes in management philosophy and practice that have the potential to reduce prisoners' suffering.

Reform efforts seem to be integral to the continuing existence of penal systems. In addition to the better known waves of 'conscience' (Rothman, 1980) in US prison history, such as the reformatory movement in the early twentieth century, individual institutions and penal systems have undertaken countless more modest projects. Change for the better has certainly occurred, particularly when education and vocational programmes were made available to inmates. But 'improvement' also contributes to the long-term viability of the prison complex; historically, projects of change intertwine with practices of exclusion and coercion that persist for generations (Foucault, 1979). Supermax, the most extreme and least humane form of contemporary confinement, raises this issue in a particularly acute form.[4] How can we do what is obviously needed for those confined in these prisons right now? And does this carry the danger that 'soft' rather than 'hard' warehousing (Toch, *see* Chapter 1) aids the perpetuation of these regimes? In this chapter I sketch out some of the implications of these questions and, despite reservations about the likelihood of their long-term implementation, outline a few practical suggestions to improve conditions for supermax prisoners.

The nature of supermax confinement

Supermaximum prisons are fortress-like facilities designed to produce regimes of separation and isolation; they may be freestanding or, more commonly, contained within larger prisons. Details of architecture and population vary, but all impose an extreme form of confinement that goes beyond the 'segregation' that has always been a necessary aspect of incarceration. Inmates are held 23 or more hours a day in single cells from which they are removed only under escort for brief showers or solitary exercise. Their lives are characterised by lack of movement, stimulation, and social contact, as well as by extreme dependence on prison staff. In some facilities the cells are windowless or have windows frosted over; lights are left on all night. Most units are noisy, although in some prisons heavy or double doors muffle sound. Inmates are cuffed, tethered, and escorted when brought out of their cells; sometimes they are shackled and searched every time they are moved. Defiant or disturbed prisoners are subjected to forcible removal from their cells ('cell extraction'), the use of pepper spray or electronic controls (tasers, electric shields, and stun belts), confinement in restraint chairs, and the imposition of 'isolation time' during which they receive sack lunches and no exercise.[5] Interactions with staff are often of the most basic parent/child kind, consisting of 'I want/You can't have' exchanges (Toch, 2001).

Personality, previous experiences, the length and conditions of confinement, the perceived fairness of the punishment (Bonta and Gendreau, 1984), and the availability of institutional and family support intersect to produce varied responses to solitude and isolation. Some supermax prisoners speak of being in a 'tomb' in which they feel numb or dead. Others describe sleep disturbances, extremes of rage or lethargy, increasing paranoia or hallucinatory experiences, and an inability to tolerate the presence of other people. Joe Giarratano, imprisoned at Virginia's Red Onion supermax, writes:

> [It requires a] tremendous amount of mental concentration . . . just to keep one's head above water. There are times, even now [after many years of confinement in various prisons] when I'm not so sure of my own grip on reality. The social isolation, greatly restricted environmental and intellectual stimulation, forced idleness, constant confinement to a small space day after day, being subjected to a constant denial of one's innate humanity and dignity – constantly being treated like an object and not a human being – the total lack of personal privacy . . . will, I suppose, take its toll on anyone . . . I must remain on guard against hallucinations, feelings of suffocation, paranoia, fear, and even rage.
>
> (McCarthy, 2000, p. 108)[6]

Some prisoners released from this form of confinement back into the general prison population or directly to the streets report that they have difficulty adjusting to life outside. In contrast, however, some prisoners describe being made stronger, or 'strong-minded,' by isolation, or insist that they prefer being alone and safe from the stress and danger of crowded general population units.

Prison officials and the media often refer to supermax as a 'prison within a prison' and to supermax prisoners as the 'worst of the worst.' They represent these facilities as necessary for incapacitation and deterrence within prison systems and as the only way to deal with predatory or out-of-control inmates. The implication is that supermax is used only for those who have committed serious crimes and that placement and lengths of stay are systematically related to the extent of criminal behaviour. But in fact, although some supermax inmates have committed serious crimes, behaviour in prison rather than criminal history (at least in theory) is the primary determinant of placement. And not all supermax prisoners are in fact being punished for serious misbehaviour in prison; they may be under protective custody, in preventive detention, or mentally ill and unable to understand or follow prison rules. Further, the fact that some prisoners harm other inmates and staff does not explain the proliferation of supermax beds over the past 25 years, or the increase in the length of supermax sentences. As Kurki and Morris put it: 'Why this splurge of money and harshness? Have prisoners become more violent, more dangerous? The data do not so suggest' (2001, p. 391). Instead, Kurki and Morris contend, popular arguments that incapacitation of difficult prisoners 'normalizes' the general population or that the presence of a supermax has a deterrent effect should be understood more as rhetoric than fact (*ibid.*, p. 391).

Because prison systems are reluctant to allow access to observers or researchers, supermax incarceration is a largely hidden aspect of the penal system as a whole. Questions about how individuals are affected or whether incapacitation actually works as advertised in reducing inmate-on-inmate violence have scarcely been addressed. More research into effects on prisoners and prison systems is certainly needed. But the larger point is that supermax prisons, however rationalised, also embody a set of assumptions and practices in which punitive individualism intersects with overwhelming power to produce an environment that is, by its very nature, inhumane.

Why there can be no 'humane' supermax

Faced with the near-impossible task of conveying their circumstances to outsiders, supermax prisoners like Joe Giarratano refer to violations of their 'innate humanity and dignity' and to the ways in which this form of confinement reduces them to the status of an 'object and not a human being.' These dehumanising effects on individuals are produced by two interconnected aspects of this form of confinement: first, the sheer physical isolation and immobility imposed by supermax and second, the social relations that flow from this form of physical deprivation. These conditions, in turn, can produce or exacerbate mental illness in prisoners, as well as give rise to extreme exercises of power on the part of staff.

The deprivation of supermax is embedded in a mechanistic operation with an overriding emphasis on efficiency and security at the expense of any individual's specific needs or desires. Surveillance is intense, and food, exercise, showers, toilet paper, and all other items are delivered – sometimes erratically or arbitrarily – based on the schedules and attitudes of staff. Prisoners are deprived of movement, daylight, darkness, predictable periods of quiet and rest, and reasonable amounts of sensory stimulation, social contact, and privacy. Inmates thus lack control over environmental and social stimulation and have few reliable means of self-soothing. Physical discomforts and scheduling uncertainties that might not trouble those living in less restricted environments take on disproportionate importance, with many prisoners describing an unrelenting sense of pressure or tension that they are unable to resolve.[7]

These extreme aspects of isolation can obscure the fact that even the supermax is a social world, however sparing and harsh its outlines. This world includes administrators and officers (guards) as well as inmates, and has features that tend to produce some kinds of social interaction and not others. Of course the most obvious of these features is the isolation of the prisoners in their small, densely walled and barricaded cells. They never have a face-to-face conversation (except for the occasional visit through thick plastic windows), are never touched (except during uses of force), and are at a more or less constant distance from others. Some prisoners become accustomed to this distance and lose tolerance for social contact.[8] Others, desperate for attention, engage in gestures such as refusing to return meal trays, or, more seriously, self-mutilation that force staff to engage. A negative, rage-ful, noisy and threatening atmosphere is typical in these environments, with few resources available to prisoners or staff to break the tension.

Perhaps the most important social feature of supermax is the overwhelming power differential between staff and inmates. The power of the staff derives most obviously from the fact that inmates are unable to group or act together, but also from inmates' extreme dependency, and from the ease with which staff can carry out operations against individuals in their cells. When overwhelming force can be brought to the door of the cell, with the back-up of pepper spray, electronic shields, restraint chairs, shackles and isolation cells, any resistance is likely to be sporadic and short-lived. This kind of architectural and structural power also has less obvious corollaries. Unlike in a general population prison, staff do not need the cooperation of the prisoners in order to manage the facility. In the absence of strong leadership or outside monitoring, this situation lends itself to abuse ranging from physical assaults on inmates (see, e.g., Human Rights Watch, 1999) to callousness and unresponsiveness to their everyday needs. Further, the security concerns expressed in the design of these units – that is, the desire to isolate inmates – tend also to produce an isolation of the entire facility. Prisoners experience this as extreme distance from the outside world, an increase in their 'reputation' for violence, or outright abandonment. Officers feel that they are alone with particularly dangerous or unworthy 'others' toward whom they can behave as they choose. Finally, while it is true that supermax prisoners are held in such a way that they are unlikely to directly harm others, this does not mean that they necessarily resign themselves to a position of utter powerlessness. Troubling if ultimately futile forms of resistance develop in these environments, such as throwing or smearing faeces, flooding cells (by stopping up the toilet), covering windows, and attempting to resist escort. Some prisoners may become obsessed with fantasies of revenge; others see 'society' as the source of their suffering and aim their revenge at targets in the world outside rather than the staff who manage their confinement (Rhodes, 2005).

Supermax conditions are directly damaging to the mental health of many prisoners, and observers report finding psychotic, delusional, severely depressed, and suicidal prisoners locked down in solitary cells (Kupers, 1999; Rhodes, 2005; Haney, 2003; Human Rights Watch, 1997). Mentally ill inmates – who make up an increasing segment of the US prison population[9] – are often unable to manage themselves under conditions of group living in general population. These prisoners accumulate multiple infractions against prison rules that send them into lock-down facilities and sometimes keep them there well beyond the time a less disturbed inmate would 'serve' for the same offence. Other prisoners, even those who do fairly well in general population, may become psychotic or develop extremely disturbed behaviour under conditions of isolation.[10] A Washington state study found that 25 to 30 per cent of supermax prisoners are mentally ill (Lovell et al., 2000). A recent case against the supermax at Boscobel, Wisconsin, was successful in removing mentally ill prisoners on the grounds that 'the decision to place a seriously mentally ill inmate at Supermax is an Eighth Amendment [against cruel and unusual punishment] violation in and of itself' regardless of whether psychiatric care is provided (Jones'El v. Berge, 164 F. Supp.2d 1096).

The two aspects of supermax confinement that have received the most attention are this presence of the mentally ill and the effect on them of 'sensory deprivation,' issues linked by the fact that sensory deprivation can lead to psychotic breakdown (Kupers, 1999; Haney, 2003). The Boscobel case was decided on the 'inappropriateness of subjecting such persons to a . . . programme that is so all encompassing and harsh' (Jones'El v. Berge, 164 F. Supp.2d 1096). However morally compelling as well as useful this argument against supermax proves to be on a case-by-case basis, we also need to keep in mind that it occurs within a larger situation. Even when mentally ill prisoners are removed, the 'strong-minded' remain. These prisoners are neither being prepared for release nor helped to manage themselves in prison. Prisoners' individual vulnerabilities are important to understanding why supermax isolation is harmful. But arguments for the rescue of the 'vulnerable' leave untouched the central problematic of these prisons, which is that they impoverish the social personhood of both prisoners and staff regardless of whether immediate ill effects can be demonstrated.

Larger contexts of supermax

Some supermax prisons are large, freestanding institutions housing several thousand inmates. But because these prisons are inevitably and necessarily embedded in the operation of the larger penal system, none are really 'free-standing.' Much that influences what happens in the planning, design and operation of a supermax has its origins elsewhere: prison overcrowding that results in fights and 'wars' among inmates; racial disproportion in the prison population as a whole, as well as racially motivated placements on the part of staff; concerns about prisoners whose 'reputations' in general population have made them difficult to place; incidents of rape or the fear of rape; popular and clinical representations of 'the worst' criminals as not only incapable of rehabilitation but also non-human (cf. Garland, 2001). Little information is available, but we can speculate that the more supermax beds are available, the more they will be used to 'solve' these problems of the larger system and society. But while supermax confinement does temporarily incapacitate, it does nothing to address systemic problems either within the system or, ultimately, in the larger community. Instead, as these prisons have become a routine (and often valorised) aspect of the penal complex, it becomes increasingly difficult for corrections departments and legislators to imagine doing without them.

In addition to being deeply embedded in larger systemic problems, the supermax is a concentrated manifestation of pervasive cultural assumptions that also underpin much normal prison operation. One of these is an over-whelming focus on notions of individual 'choice' and autonomy. Inmates are assumed to be making personal choices that are almost entirely free of contextual constraints; 'behaviour,' many prison workers and legislators insist, should be capable of correction through punishments that make 'choices' as clear as possible. This means prisoners in supermax can be seen to have 'chosen' to be there and to need nothing other than ample solitary time to consider the consequences of their actions. Despite the routinised nature of much of the daily operation of supermax both staff and inmates are engaged in a struggle over these fundamental issues of agency and intentionality. Do disturbed inmates, for example, 'intend' their behaviour?[11] Is it possible to allow for environmental influences – such as the effects of isolation – or are such allowances a dangerous slide into 'softness?' Is an officer's or an inmate's sense of himself as a man compromised by negotiation of any kind?[12] Such framings of the relation between individual and society are embedded, as Garland suggests, in a late modern system of exile in which '"our" security [is seen to] depend upon "their" control' (*ibid.*, p. 182).

Ameliorating supermax confinement

Is there, then, a harm-reduction strategy that can address at least some of the suffering produced by routine supermax confinement? I think the answer is a qualified yes. Precisely because much of the daily misery of supermax rests in the malign intersection of isolation with discomfort and indignity, relatively small changes can make a significant difference to prisoners. At the same time, these kinds of changes are in no way an answer to the larger issues raised by the existence of these prisons. Nor, despite their seeming obviousness, are they easy to implement. Much in the current correctional landscape militates against the kinds of leadership, changes in attitude, and shifts in policy needed to make these changes.[13]

Planning and design

Perhaps the most important step toward ameliorating supermax confinement is not to build these facilities in the first place. A former corrections official recommends that:

> An agency should carefully consider the number of extended control beds that are or will be needed . . . overbuilding . . . capacity . . . may cause problems operationally and legally as the agency attempts to house inmates in an extended control environment who do not require that level of custody or security.
>
> (Riveland, 1999, p.19)

'Overbuilt capacity' makes it too easy for general population units to send inmates into supermax, and too easy for supermax staff to keep them. And no matter how many beds are made available, they never seem 'enough' from the perspective of prison staff struggling with overcrowded general population conditions. Pressure from prison staff, concerns about risk and litigation, and the enthusiasm of architecture, building, and equipment firms (and thus, legislators) for new construction should therefore be weighed against the long-term effects of increasing reliance on lock-down capacity.

When new facilities are built or old ones renovated, equally careful attention should be given from the beginning to creating the least restrictive and harmful environment. Prisoners are greatly affected by details of design that may seem trivial to planners, such as the difference between 'natural light' provided through a clerestory far from an inmate's line of vision and a window through which he can actually see the sky. Other important details include cell interior and door design, exercise facilities, temperature regulation, and adequate break rooms and outdoor access for staff.

Admission and release

Supermax units fill with ease and empty with difficulty. Because they are used, as I've described, to address problems not being resolved elsewhere in the system, the process of admission tends to be efficient and local. In some institutions, staff of general population units expect their supermax counterparts to provide unquestioned respite from 'difficult' or 'nuisance' inmates. The process of release, on the other hand, may depend on decisions by officials and administrators at several levels, many with reason to be highly risk-averse. Finding the right balance of local and system-wide decision-making on admission and release is not easy; overly rigid policies prevent local administrators from responding to situations only they may understand (such as, for instance, the mental deterioration of a prisoner) while, on the other hand, lack of oversight may result in punitive and unnecessary – or years-long – supermax sentences for inmates with bad reputations or other problems. Admission practices also require oversight and balance regarding over-long sentences in general, racial/ethnic disproportion, and the use of extreme punitive measures such as isolation time. Policies on release should include frequent review and hearings (ideally, with an outside observer present), transitional housing and programmes for inmates who have been under supermax confinement for long periods or who have behavioural problems, and no release directly to the streets. In addition to these measures for all prisoners, the mentally ill should be removed from supermax confinement, and solutions sought for inmates who fall between the cracks of mental illness and 'bad behaviour.'

Attention to prisoners

Prisoners locked into isolation are deprived of the means to deal with even the most basic aspects of their lives. For example, a prisoner may be unable to reach his family during the brief yard time in which he has access to a phone. At the same time, supermax units are designed so that officers can avoid contact with inmates – hurrying past their cells, ignoring kites (notes) or shouts for help, failing to provide information about their status or prospects for release. Such contact as exists may be perfunctory or demeaning. Yet this is one aspect of these prisons that can be altered dramatically without any additional resources or policy changes. A 'walk-through' or 'tier walk' is the practice of staff – including top administrators – going regularly from cell to cell, listening and responding to each prisoner as needed. During a tier walk prisoners are able to complain about conditions, inquire about their release status, and make requests for basic items. Mental and physical health problems, problems with meal service, and breakdowns in unit security and maintenance are revealed to supervisors and become harder to brush aside. This simple change brings higher level staff onto a unit, keeps unit staff informed of prisoners' everyday frustrations, and creates pressure on officers to handle requests and problems as they come up. Gary Jones, an administrator who instituted tier walks in a troubled Washington State supermax, writes that:

After a couple of months, all supervisors and unit managers were attending walk-throughs . . . Supervisors and managers began seeing less paperwork to respond to. Grievances were nearly non-existent because we could handle the problem much more quickly . . . Infraction behaviour was reduced by 50 per cent in the first six months. Hundreds of grievances that lay on my desk when I started at the unit were gone within six months, and none replaced them. The thousands of dollars in damages to the unit had been reduced to zero during the first six months.

(Jones, 2005)

Waiting periods and negotiations before cell extractions (barring emergencies) can also significantly reduce violence and distress in these facilities. Jones writes of his experience in changing the previous regime of precipitous and aggressive cell extraction that ' . . . all controlled uses of force had a cause and effect in these units . . . staff actions or inaction . . . precipitated the event' (*ibid.*, 2005). Other, similarly straightforward practices include consistent attention to unit cleanliness and officer scheduling, and retaining well-trained mental health staff with good access to whatever psychiatric facilities are available in the system as a whole. Unfortunately, none of these things is easily accomplished, in part because the cultural assumptions I've discussed make it difficult to 'soften' these regimes.

Although better than nothing, television, visiting booths, written courses, and other measures to address sensory deprivation or simply to keep inmates occupied do not address the scope of social isolation in supermax nor the kinds of socialisation and transition programmes many prisoners need. For some, especially those ready and waiting for release, carefully planned contact with other inmates in the form of congregate classes and exercise should be developed.

Attention to staff

Supermax prisons are problematic as working environments in ways that to some extent parallel their effect on prisoners. Staff conduct the mechanical, repetitive tasks of counting, escorting, surveillance, and meal delivery in an isolated, harsh environment, often with little support from administrators. Many are from the rural areas in which these prisons are built, with little understanding of or empathy for urban prisoners. The behaviour and attitudes of staff should be addressed not only with adequate training and no-tolerance policies on abuse, but also by creating acceptable and respectful ways for them to interact with prisoners. In addition, staff need adequate breaks during the work day, relief-time away from the unit, and opportunities to communicate with administrators and with staff working other shifts. Increasing workers' sense of safety and renovating ageing infrastructure can also improve treatment of inmates.

Conclusion

The proliferation of supermax prisons amounts to the development, at the national and now international levels, of an institutional form designed for a semi-permanent or permanent state of profound social exclusion (Agamben,

1998). Over the past 30 years political, popular, and clinical representations of criminality, as well as a series of 'moral panics' (Tonry, 2004), have contributed to the dehumanising of prisoners in public discourse. The prison has become a 'kind of reservation, a quarantine zone' intended purely to segregate (Garland, 2001, p. 178). The supermax is at the extreme end of this zone, providing the criminal justice system with the option of semi-permanent lock-down, and intensifying and normalising the sense that quarantine is the 'natural' response to social disorder. During this same time period, relatively little attention has gone into the issue of reinclusion – of how quarantined individuals might be helped with the transition out of prison and made part of the social fabric again. With their inflexible design and aura of stability, supermax prisons thus reinforce the current rejection of rehabilitation. Expensive to build but so specialised that they are useless for any other purpose, they seem likely to persist into the near-distant future.

Perhaps in a different political and economic landscape the possibility of dismantling these prisons and rethinking necessary levels of segregation will find some purchase. We live, however, in 'an untidy, thoroughly implicating "second best world"' (Redfield, 2005, quoting Terry, 2002). 'The challenge,' as Davis notes, ' . . . is to do the work that will create more humane, habitable environments for people in prison without bolstering the permanence of the prison system' (Davis, 2003, p. 103). The suggestions I have made here – echoing those of other observers and participants in the prison system – are obvious but minimal responses to the situation of supermax confinement. Further, they hold together contradictions, such as providing interaction from the same people doing the confining, that hold the seeds of their own unravelling. Supermax prisons can be made more habitable but, as a supermax administrator invested in changing his unit put it, 'We do not get our full humanity until these people go out into a normal situation' (Rhodes, 2004, p. 209).

References

Agamben G (1998) (D Heller-Roazen, trans.) *Homo Sacer: sovereign power and bare life*. Stanford University Press, Stanford, CA.

Bonta J and Gendreau P (1984) Solitary confinement is not cruel and unusual punishment: people sometimes are! *Canadian Journal of Criminology*. **26**: 467–8.

Bureau of Justice Statistics (2003). www.ojp.usdoj.gov/bjs/correct.htm#findings.

Camp C and Camp G (eds) (2000) *The Corrections Yearbook 2000: adult corrections*. Criminal Justice Institute, Middleton, CT.

Caplow T and Simon J (1999) Understanding prison policy and population trends. In: M Tonry and J Petersilia. *Prisons*. University of Chicago Press, Chicago, IL.

Davis AY (2003) *Are Prisons Obsolete?* Seven Stories Press, New York, NY.

Foucault M (1979) *Discipline and Punish: the birth of the prison*. Vintage, New York, NY.

Garland D (2001) *The Culture of Control: crime and social order in contemporary society*. University of Chicago Press, Chicago, IL.

Haney C (2003) Mental Health Issues in Long-term Solitary and 'Supermax' Confinement. *Crime and Delinquency*. **49**(1): 124-56.

Human Rights Watch (1997) *Cold Storage: super-maximum security confinement in Indiana.* Human Rights Watch, New York, NY.

Human Rights Watch (1999) *Red Onion State Prison: super-maximum confinement in Virginia.* Human Rights Watch, New York, NY.

Jemelka R, Turpin E and Chiles JA (1989) The mentally ill in prisons: a review. *Hospital and Community Psychiatry.* **40**: 481–5.

Jones' El v Berge, 164F Supppld. 1096 (WD Wis. 2001) United States District Court for the Western District of Wisconsin. 10 October 2001. www.gele.org/law/2002JBAPR/jvb.html.

Jones G (2005) Statement of Gary D. Jones. Commission on Safety and Abuse in America's Prisons, Public Hearing 2. www.prisoncommission.org/public_hearing_2.asp.

Kupers T (1999) *Prison Madness: the mental health crisis behind bars and what we can do about it.* Jossey-Bass, San Francisco, CA.

Kurki L and Morris N (2001) The purposes, practices and problems of supermax prisons. In: Tonry M (ed) *Crime and Justice: a review of research.* University of Chicago Press, Chicago, IL.

Lakoff G (1999) *Moral Politics: how liberals and conservatives think* (2e). Chicago University Press, Chicago, IL.

Lovell D, Cloyes K, David GA and Rhodes LA (2000) Who lives in supermaximum custody?: A Washington State study. *Federal Probation.* **61**(3): 40–45.

McCarthy C (2000) *A governor's doubt of a man's guilt isn't enough in Virginia.* Joseph Giarratano. National Catholic reporter. 15 September.

National Institute of Corrections (1997) *Supermax Housing: A survey of current practice.* US Department of Justice, Longmint.

Redfield P (2005) Doctors, borders and life in crisis. *Cultural Anthropology.* **20**(3): 328–61.

Rhodes LA (2004) *Total Confinement: madness and reason in the maximum security prison.* University of California Press, Berkeley, CA.

Rhodes LA (2005) Changing the subject: conversation in supermax. *Cultural Anthropology.* **20**(3): 388–411.

Riveland C (1999) *Supermax Prisons: overview and general considerations.* National Institute of Corrections, US Department of Justice. US Department of Justice, Washington, DC.

Rothman DJ (1980) *Conscience and Convenience: the asylum and its alternatives in progressive America.* Little, Brown, Boston, MA.

Terry F (2002) *Condemned to Repeat? The Paradox of Humanitarian Action.* Cornell University Press, Ithaca, NY.

Toch H (2001) The Life of Lifers: Wolfgang's inquiry into the prison adjustment of homicide offenders. In: RA Silverman (ed) *Marvin E. Wolfgang, Crime and Justice at the Millennium: Essays by and in Honor of Marvin E. Wolfgang.* Kluwer, Boston, MA.

Tonry, M (2004) *Thinking about Crime: sense and sensibility in American penal culture.* Oxford University Press, Oxford.

Ward DA and Werlich TG (2003) Alcatraz and Marion: evaluating super-maximum custody. *Punishment and Society.* **5**(1): 53–75.

Notes

1 The US prison population is now over two million (Bureau of Justice Statistics 2003). Although the rate of expansion has slowed, and sentencing policies are changing in some states, the system continues to grow. Exact figures are not

available, but some 20 to 40 000 people may now be confined in supermax facilities, and new ones continue to be built. The most recent account of supermax construction in the United States is a report by the National Institute of Corrections compiled in 1997 (NIC, 1997). See also Riveland, 1999; Rhodes, 2004; Camp and Camp, 2000). Riveland notes one of the difficulties in determining the number of supermax facilities: 'jurisdictions do not share a common definition of supermax due to their differing needs, classification criteria and methods, and operational considerations (Riveland, 1999, p. 3). The supermax model has expanded beyond the United States to the United Kingdom, Turkey, Iraq, South Africa and elsewhere.

2 There are five main sources of information on supermax confinement: reports from human rights groups; prisoners' accounts; court documents; accounts based on research within prison systems; and statistical information from which one can try to deduce the population composition of these prisons. This article draws on these sources, on my ethnographic account of maximum security prisons in Washington State, and on a reform effort in one Washington prison (Rhodes, 2004, pp. 191–228; Jones, 2005). I also draw on a larger Washington State study conducted between 1999 and 2002 as part of a University of Washington/Department of Correction Mental Health Collaboration in which I and my colleagues (David Allen, David Lovell, Kristen Cloyes and Cheryl Cooke) interviewed 97 randomly selected inmates and 40 staff in three of the state's control units (Lovell et al., 2000; Rhodes, 2004; 2005). Unless otherwise indicated the comments of prisoners and staff given here are from my ethnographic notes or from these interviews; I studied male-only prisons and use the masculine pronoun here. It is important to note that the United States has considerable variation from state to state, as well as at the federal level, in how these prisons are filled and managed. One significant issue is whether supermax inmates are held indefinitely under 'preventive detention' for 'gang-related' activities. Washington State does not have an official policy of preventive detention. For a discussion of differences in prison philosophy and management between the United States and Europe, see Kurki and Morris (2001, pp. 415–17).

3 The question of what has driven the development of the massive US prison complex is beyond the scope of this chapter. An individualistic and punitive orientation, an increasingly militarised criminal justice system, and the economic pressures of neoliberalism and globalization are some of the contributing factors (Rhodes, 2004; Garland, 2001; Caplow and Simon, 1999; Kurki and Morris, 2001).

4 Supermax might perhaps more properly be called the most extreme publicly legitimised form of late modern confinement; detention camps and other concealed prisons are further out on the continuum of extreme practices.

5 See Kurki and Morris (2001) and Rhodes (2004) for more detailed descriptions of the internal operations and atmosphere of supermax.

6 Other prisoner accounts of supermax are available and make similar points. I chose this one as my example here because Giarratano writes of himself as someone with perhaps more inner resources than many prisoners. Yet it is a struggle for him to withstand supermax conditions.

7 Most supermax prisons operate on a behavioural system consisting of 'levels' or 'steps.' At the lowest level, either upon admission or as a result of poor 'behaviour,' inmates may be given nothing but a Bible or Koran; higher levels (better 'behaviour') result in access to radio, television, more reading materials, and other privileges. While these systems may alleviate the worst conditions of solitary confinement, they can also reinforce punitive and individualistic approaches that divorce 'behaviour' from its context and effect an imaginary transfer of agency to the prisoner.

Whether or not they change prisoners' behaviour once released is unknown, though see Ward and Werlich for an argument that they do (2003).

8 I have written elsewhere about the kind of conversations that are possible among supermax inmates in some of these prisons (Rhodes, 2005).

9 Jemelka *et al.*, (1989) found that at least 10 to 15 per cent of admissions to Washington State prisons meet clinical criteria for serious mental illness.

10 The extent to which this occurs in the absence of previous vulnerabilities is unclear; no longitudinal research has been done on the effects of supermax confinement on either mentally ill or non-mentally ill inmates.

11 Ironically, the issue of choice and intention recurs at the level of administrative intention. The authors of *Cold Storage* say, for example, that although 'we do not believe that the Indiana DOC has the specific intent of tormenting mentally ill prisoners . . . [however] the housing of these prisoners in supermax units represents a serious and indefensible failure to provide adequate psychiatric treatment and facilities' (1997, p. 12).

12 See Lakoff (1999) on the language of the larger political landscape within which this logic operates.

13 For a more expansive and ethnographically grounded discussion, see Rhodes (2005); for more detailed recommendations see, especially, Riveland (1999) and Human Rights Watch (1997).

Chapter 8

The UK Prison Service Close Supervision Centres

Mark Morris

For the last decade, an innovative structure for the management of the 30 or 40 most dangerous and disruptive prisoners in the UK prison population of over 75 000 has been evolving, known as the Close Supervision Centre – or CSC system. In this paper I hope to describe these units by looking briefly at their historical context and evolution, by making an attempt to describe the diverse combination of difficulties that they try to manage and by looking at the ideological framework on which they are based.

The historical context

Traditionally, the management of very difficult prisoners has been a pragmatic affair between governors of prisons. Prior to the development of managerialism in the public services and an increase in the central managerial authority of 'headquarters', individual prison governors seem to have been relatively autonomous in the management of their prisons. The traditional method, therefore, for managing difficult prisoners must have grown out of this; one governor would have a prisoner who had burnt out the staff, whom they needed a break from; the governor of a colleague prison would have someone with a similar profile, and the two governors would 'swap' prisoners, on the grounds that a change was as good as a rest. It is often the case that difficult people spiral into a vicious circle with their carers, such that a fresh team bring a genuine improvement, a new start that can sometimes be sustained. More often the same problems emerge in the new setting, but even so, for the sake of both prisoner and staff, the move can be justified on the grounds of the 'honeymoon' period of respite.

With the increasing national coordinating function of the central prison authority, these informal 'swaps' of prisoners developed into a system known to staff as the 'Continuous Assessment System' (CAS), where prisoners would be moved periodically between the intensive management (segregation) units of the different prisons; in very extreme cases as often as every six weeks. This strategy was adopted to maximise the beneficial effect of a new team with a prisoner. The new team would know that they would only be looking after a prisoner for a set time, and therefore would be more happy to agree to take the prisoner, and so it managed the deleterious effects on staff and morale that these people can have when they are in a destructive phase. Prisoners dubbed this the 'merry-go-round'; the difficulties were clear to see: that other than those running the system at headquarters, there was little continuity of care, and there was not time for the staff in the different units to get to know the person, which is often the most important aspect of interpersonal prison-craft and the management of difficult people.

In the early 1990s, influenced by the success of the Special Unit in Barlinnie Prison, several special units were set up across the country. The hypothesis was that very difficult people might become increasingly difficult as the regime within which they were managed became more austere and securely structured. The evidence from the Barlinnie Unit was that, given more freedom and a more relaxed regime, the number of assaults on staff and other disturbances reduced. Unfortunately, as with the Barlinnie unit, concerns about security and one or two worrying incidents illustrated that there was serious potential for this group of people to utilise the reduction in secure restriction manipulatively. Given the high profile and violent and disruptive potential of the individuals there could be catastrophic consequences. The Close Supervision Centre (CSC) system was conceived in the discussions following these difficulties, to try to combine the success that accrued from the format of intensively staffing centrally coordinated specialist units with specially trained personnel, with a more prison and security-type emphasis. The new structure was underpinned by a new prison rule, 'Rule 46' – complementary to 'Rule 45' which governs the process of segregation of violent and disruptive prisoners. Rule 46 and the CSC system was a national system for highly disruptive prisoners requiring central oversight and management.

The overall managerial structure of the CSC system has remained constant, although over the years, there have been developments in the culture of practice and conceptualisation of the task, and in the geographical units involved. The administration of Rule 46 takes place in a monthly meeting notionally chaired by the Home Secretary but in practice by his designate, the director of the high-security prisons or his nominee, i.e. a senior and centrally involved prison service executive. Technically, each prisoner is detained under Rule 46 for a month, and their detention is renewed at this monthly meeting, attended by the CSC unit staff from across the country. At the outset, a research and evaluation project was commissioned that reported after the first few years, and an independent oversight group comprising senior academics and clinicians was established to monitor the work, partly given the human rights implications and other possible controversies.

The three phases of CSC development

CSC practice and conceptualisation of task can be divided into three phases over the years.

Phase 1

Phase 1 seems to have had similarities to the UK prison service 'incentives and earned privileges' structure that was being developed at the same time. Broadly, it comprised a rewards system, where responsible behaviour and an absence of adverse events leads to enhanced privileges and regimes. Geographically, the CSC system comprised five units across two geographical sites, one in Woodhill Prison in Milton Keynes, and the other in Durham Prison. Passage through the CSC was conceived of as progression through three different stages – the first being 'A wing' Woodhill, with availability of rehabilitation and other activities reduced because of the need for a highly structured and safe regime; the second being 'B wing' Woodhill, where there was more opportunity for rehabilitative activities as prisoners had demon-strated some evidence of responsible and safe behaviour such that the risks that they presented had been reduced somewhat. The third was 'G wing' Durham, conceived of as a rehabilitative unit, preparing prisoners for return to normal prison location. In addition to these three phased progressive units, there was 'I wing' Durham, which was for prisoners with clearer psychiatric difficulties requiring specialist support, and who were not easily fitted into the progressive model; and there was 'D wing' Woodhill – conceived of as the CSC intensive care unit for prisoners presenting an exceptionally high risk, but dubbed by prisoners as the 'CSC seg.' or the 'superseg.' (Segregation Unit).

This Phase 1 model did have its successes, notably in demonstrating that the model of centralised management and coordination of the most difficult prisoners in specialist units was effective, and that the managerial and legal underpinning was robust, but within the Woodhill unit some difficulties emerged. The motivation is unclear, but it is possible that a number of prisoners recognised the progressive nature of the CSC's structure, and decided to fight it by amplifying their disruptive and difficult behaviour. As a consequence, for a period, there were a number of prisoners who required treatment in the D wing Woodhill intensive care unit. One of the most dangerous aspects of these prisoners is their ability to incite and coordinate unrest, and it is probable that there was some organisation amongst the prisoner group involved in these difficulties. Reflection on these difficulties, along with recommendations from a contiguous Inspectorate Thematic Review (HMIP, 1999) seems to have contributed to the development of the 'phase' model.

Phase 2

Phase 2 combined the extension of the system geographically with the development of individualised care planning. The extension of the system geographically involved firstly a new unit in Wakefield Prison that would work with long-term exceptionally high-risk prisoners; secondly a four-bed dedicated unit in Long Lartin prison in Evesham within its intensive treat-ment unit; and thirdly up to two cells in the segregation units of the high-security prisons would be available for CSC prisoners under rule 46 for respite stays. These facilities enhanced ability to provide individualised packages of care by separating groups of prisoners who collectively conspired to undermine their progress and the structure of the service, as well as increasing the flexibility of the system to respond to individual prisoners' needs, for example, those with long-term and enduring levels of risk.

The individualised care planning structure was modelled on the National Health Service Care Programme Approach, which structures psychiatric care in the UK through a process of regular multidisciplinary reviews of identified treatment targets towards a particular rehabilitative trajectory, in which the subject is a participant. The development of these 'Care and Management' meetings and plans for all of the prisoners in the system was highly effective in moving from a 'one size fits all' approach to management, to each person having a clear and individualised understanding of what needed to happen for them to make progress, and having a sense of what a progressive path might be. Allied to this was the further development of the structure of admission to the CSC system – the previously mentioned detention under Rule 46. The assessment procedure that was developed involved multidisciplinary assessment and case conferencing that would recommend to the CSC management committee how to proceed. The multidisciplinary assessments included a psychiatric history and evaluation, a psychological history involving various empirical risk assessment tools, and a full historical risk evaluation and assessment carried out by probation and custodial staff. The significance of a move from a prison control culture of management to a multidisciplinary care planning type of approach cannot be over-emphasised, both in the improvement in the legitimacy of management decisions that have been debated by a multidisciplinary group, and in the development of a sense of a team sharing the struggle to tackle the problems posed.

Phase 3

The development of Phase 3 of the CSC units seems to have been driven in part by contextual changes, including, on the one hand, the international academic focus on treatment programmes for highly psychopathic individuals, mirrored in the UK with the Dangerous and Severe Personality Disorder (DSPD) treatment proposals (Home Office/DoH, 1999), and, on the other, the UK government's NHS Plan (DoH, 2000) identifying prison mental health care as a development priority, which has had the effect of greatly improving the provision and availability of psychiatric opinion and management for mentally disordered offenders in prison. Changes in the geographical units have included the closure of the rehabilitation unit in G wing Durham, whose role had waned following the development of an individualised approach to management rather than a process one; and the transfer of the psychiatric special needs unit from Durham I wing to Whitemoor – consequent on the re-rolling of Durham as a community rather than a high security prison.

The heart of the CSC Phase 3 development is the incorporation of thinking and therapeutic conceptualisation and strategies from Wong and Gordon's 'Violence Reduction Programme' (VRP) (Wong and Gordon, 2003). Structurally, this has involved the creation of a dedicated unit where the programme is run in E wing Woodhill. Culturally, it has involved the re-conceptualisation of the work of the CSC system as the UK Prison Services violence reduction programme. Particularly helpful in providing a context for face-to-face work with prisoners is the notion of phases of treatment – that it is essential for therapeutic intervention to be effective that prisoners realise that they have a problem that they need to tackle; that frequently prisoners do not see themselves as contributors to their problems, and that this recognition is a highly significant treatment target; that following this, there is an interactive process of understanding the nature of their difficulty; and that subsequent to this, there is the opportunity for a skills acquisition model of developing alternative strategies to violent behaviour.

Allied to the development of a specific VRP treatment unit and development of a CSC-wide conceptualisation of the work as being about violence reduction, there has been the development of a specific and specialised forensic mental heath collaborative for prisoners in the CSC. The collaborative comprises local forensic psychiatry services working together to enable the geographically dispersed CSC units to function as a whole, with shared standards and continuity of care.

Defining the problem

Traditionally, prison services are the subject of criticism, either for being too brutal, with concerns for the human rights of prisoners, or for being too soft, and too expensive. One might take a conceptual leap in firstly redefining the task of prisons primarily as providing containment for people with varying degrees of psychopathic or antisocial personality disorder, and secondly that characteristic of such difficult personalities when more severe (as found in the longer-term prison population) is the creation of chaos, anarchy and violence. From this perspective, the levels and frequency of such chaos, anarchy and violence within the prisons with the high concentration of such people and their close proximity of living conditions speaks to the effectiveness of prison structures and regimes to manage them.

Recently, there have been efforts to identify and define particular characteristics of treatment packages effective for personality-disordered patients. Essential are the factors of positive reinforcement of pro-social (as opposed to antisocial) behaviour, structure and consistency. The culture and structure of the UK prison service provides this, with its clear set of rules, its system of privileges for good behaviour and its quasi-judicial punishments for transgressions.

While this structure, consistently and rigorously applied, is effective for the majority, some cannot be contained, and require more intensive management, as well as being segregated from other prisoners in view of their disruptive potential. In the prison's segregation or intensive management unit, the principles of reward and rigour are applied more thoroughly, with more intensive staffing and engagement with individual prisoners by members of the prison management team to try to pull them back into more reasonable behaviour. This tiered structure of management contains the vast majority of prisoners, and while compliance may not be achieved over months or even years, their disruptive potential is contained. The CSC system and its predecessors are specifically targeted at the group that cannot be contained by this structure – who manage to overwhelm the structures of the segregation/intensive management unit that they have been allocated to.

Situations where standard prison structures can be overwhelmed seem to be as follows: firstly, management of a prisoner's extreme degree of violence, in terms of the pure ferocity of the antisocial and violent activity, or where a prisoner has killed or nearly killed while in custody; secondly, where the violence is at an organisational level – such violence is often psychological. Each of these will be explored in turn.

The first category of physically violent prisoners which might require transfer to the CSC system are those who need specialised management out of pure ferocity. There are two aspects to the 'ferocity'-type prisoners. Their fight is actively directed at the prison officers, and it is of an extreme nature. There are many apocryphal stories of aggressive men managing to evacuate enraged and violent feelings in various ways. Freud at one point characterised instinctual drives as having a 'hydraulic' quality, namely that there was pressure that simply needed to be let out (Freud, 1936). For some prisoners, the prison system or staff become the object of this evacuation – the target for all of their rage and violence. It seems that many more manage to redirect their rage and aggression into internal inter-prisoner 'landing politics' – so that there will be antipathies and at times fights between prisoners. There is, of course, an underlying antipathy in general for the 'screws' – the prison officers, and at times, on impulse, or following a confrontation perhaps about a rule that a prisoner has transgressed, a prison officer might be assaulted; but this animosity is different from those prisoners who actually focus their hatred and animosity at the prison staff, and go out of their way to precipitate violent confrontations.

Such prisoners usually end up being managed on the intensive management or segregation units, where the triad of close managerial oversight, intensive staffing and specialised risk management procedures contain the risks that such patients pose. However, for some prisoners, the level and degree of their violence enables them to break through this managerial matrix, such that one or more members of staff are seriously injured in an incident, or such that the level of intensity of threat itself becomes problematic. Such a situation over a long period of time can become very demoralising for staff, leading to burnout such that it has to be managed by the transfer of the prisoner to another facility, until the prisoner exhausts the new team. 'Ferocity' prisoners who move to the CSC will have been moved between various prisons, and there will come a point when there is nowhere else to send them.

The second group of physically violent prisoners are those who have been involved in a very serious incident, such as a killing, in prison. There are two factors that argue for the more specialist management of those who kill in prison, firstly the human rights and duty of care to the rest of the prison population who are at risk from the individual, and secondly the escalation of risk that killing in a custodial setting indicates. While it is true that UK prison settings can at times be violent places, and that bullying and assaults between prisoners do take place, there is an argument that these levels are low, given the twin factors of large numbers of dysfunctional and violent men that are managed in the prison setting, and given their close proximity of living. As mentioned above, it would appear that the consistency of management, the clarity of rules and structure – of reinforcements of good behaviour and the punishment of bad – reduce the potential levels of violence within a prison setting. Therefore, violent offences carried out within a prison structure denote a more severe level of pathology and risk than would an equivalent incident in the community. Prisoners who have killed or very seriously injured in prison therefore identify themselves as high-risk individuals in spite of the close level of supervision that is available in a prison setting, and in particular they represent a very high risk to their fellow prisoners, so there is an overriding duty of care to the rest of the prison population to manage them safely.

The other group of prisoners are those who are difficult to manage because of their organisational violence or disruption. In my view, it is these prisoners who present the greatest challenge to services, because whereas physical violence can be managed with physical structures and the restriction of freedom and regime, psychological and organisational violence attacks and undermines the managerial structures, strategies and personnel of the organisation attempting to manage them. Normal prison environments and their intensive management/segregation units are much more prone to being unable to manage prisoners who make a concerted organisationally violent attack than those making physical attacks, which they are geared up to work with.

Organisational violence

Organisational violence can be defined as an act that causes disruption to the organisation's functioning. It comprises three main elements: psychological violence, incitement and administrative challenge. Psychological violence saps the strength of staff working with the individual, and there are various ways that this can be achieved, usually by targeting an individual and intimidating them by threat of physical violence, complaint or litigation; by actual complaint and litigation; by conditioning and by sexual, racial or other personal abuse; or by revealing traumatising details of previous offending, violent or sexual fantasies. A frequent form of protest has been the smearing of faeces, or more recently threats to throw HIV positive blood or urine at staff. Arguably, the main impact of these threats and behaviours is psychological, with fear of development of disease and the creation of an unpleasant working environment.

Incitement of other prisoners to enact antisocial acts is a particularly high-risk activity, illustrated by the difference between a single individual becoming violent to staff, and an individual inciting a prison riot. The ability to incite others to antisocial activity requires intelligence, sensitivity to the personality and attitudes of the person being incited, and manipulativeness. Interestingly, these psychological characteristics and competencies are very similar to the characteristics of effective managerial leadership. It would appear that both managers and those with the ability to incite can motivate others to do their business. The difference lies in the psychopathic element, in that incitement in the interests of organisational violence would have an antisocial, disruptive and destructive motivation, whereas the former would be more pro-social and creative.

The third component of organisational violence is administrative challenge. At an everyday level, a challenge to the administration of the organisation might be refusal to come in from exercise, or refusal to participate in care and rehabilitative planning meetings; at an intermediate level it might be the frequent pursuit of vexatious complaints with the effect of tying up large amounts of managerial time, reducing organisational effectiveness; at a more extreme level it might be the launching of judicial reviews of the legitimacy of the CSC Rule 46 structure, or other aspects of management. Effective organisational violence requires a degree of intelligence and sophistication about the organisation's policies, procedures and operating standards, in order to be able to challenge when things are not carried out to the letter, and to be able to instruct legal advisers effectively, or construct effective complaints. Again, these aspects of functioning are similar to those required by effective managers operating in a bureaucratic organisational structure, and again, the difference between the organisationally violent individual and the effective manager will be the destructive antisocial versus creative pro-social motivation.

In the process of administrative challenge as a component of organisational violence, prisoners can abuse their fundamental rights. For example, it is absolutely essential that people detained by the state have full access to the independent investigation and evaluation of their complaints, and that they have full access to legal advice and representation in order to ensure the maintenance of their human rights and dignity. However, as with all things, they can be used appropriately, or they can be abused by being used in the service of organisational disruption rather than truly achieving justice. At times, this issue can cause confusion.

Values-based treatment and management

The specific developments in treatment approaches by the CSC have been mentioned above in discussion of the historical development of the service. In a sense, these approaches, however, are secondary to a more important set of guiding principles relating to working with this client group. I have argued that the difficulties this group of people present transcend the more straightforward tasks of managing the various physical risks, and that in addition they have ways of attacking and undermining the personnel and structure of the organisation managing them. These more insidious attacks frequently cannot be contained by the managerial policies and processes, and challenge the organisation's meta-level attitudes and functions. These attacks have the potential to (and frequently do) lay bare the basic values and practices of the containing organisation by stripping away any obfuscatory managerial rhetoric. As a consequence, a starting point in the management of these patients is to rigorously establish a group of legitimate values on which to base the work.

With this group of people who have a destructive motivation (as described above) and capacity (with their appropriate human rights-based legal support) to challenge the fundamental structures of management, it is necessary to be clear about the absolute basics of the organisation's functioning – namely its values. Furthermore, given the ferocity of administrative challenge that is mounted, these values need not only to be espoused but practised, owned and reflected in operational practice. What is described below is an attempt to articulate some of these values as I understood them operating within the CSC. Briefly they comprise: the active sustenance of the network; senior managerial oversight of legitimate structures; team functioning and staff support; the maintenance of a rehabilitative focus; and maintaining openness of process and respect for individuals. I shall look at each of these in turn.

Core values of the system

Network

As described above, the CSC system comprises a set of geographically separate units conceived as a single 'unit'. Traditionally, there are rivalries between different establishments, and given the difficult people being managed by the CSC there is potential for this to be amplified considerably by prisoners' attempts to undermine the different units working together by splitting them and creating enmities. Because of these factors, it is essential that the network of different units has the regular opportunity to meet and exchange views – for example, if prisoner A reports that he was treated in such-and-such a way in unit X, and therefore is complaining that he should have this matched in unit Y, the managers of X and Y need to be able to get together to establish the truth of the claims and forge a way forward. The first value, therefore, is that the system needs to work as a true network, rather than one simply on paper. This is achieved by monthly meetings where all the client-prisoners are discussed and their management for the subsequent month is agreed, which is attended by all of the managers of the units making up the network. In addition, at a strategic level, there are quarterly meetings of the governors of the prisons where issues can be thrashed out. The maintenance of this true network establishes a knowledge of all of the prisoner group across all of the nodes of the network, in addition to personal relationships between the different managers, who are more likely to approach each other direct by phone when faced with problems about a particular prisoner. It also establishes a firm relation between the different nodes of the network and the centre, and enhances continuity of care should people need to move from one to another.

Senior management oversight

The second value is the senior managerial oversight of legitimate structures. Characteristically, prisoners adept at administrative challenge refuse to discuss their complaints with more junior managers, being contemptuous of this, and demanding to see the most senior manager available. Frequently, in addition, they legitimately deconstruct the response to a complaint that they have been given by a more junior manager such that the query is passed up the managerial line anyway, finding its way to the desk of the most senior manger available. This has the effect of amplifying the contempt such prisoners have for their closest managers, with whom they could be working most closely, and of demoralising and undermining the junior managers' authority. The way out of this conundrum is twofold: firstly, to recognise the fact that these prisoners have the capacity to escalate their demands to the highest levels of authority, and to have oversight by these higher levels of their management and progress; secondly, to have a robust managerial and authority structure – in short, one that requires the legitimate exhaustion of the more junior managerial level prior to appeal to the higher level. Prisoners need to take issues up through the correct structures and tiers of management. A senior manager 'collared' by a prisoner about a day-to-day issue would refer the prisoner back down to the tier of management appropriate to deal with it rather than take it on themselves initially. If in good faith the issue can not be dealt with at the lowest level, then the issue would be addressed at the next lowest level. Eventually the 'collared' manager might once again have to address the issue, but only after legitimately the tiers of management below have been unable to resolve the issue. Essentially, this value is about respecting the legitimacy of tiers of managerial structure, and senior managers genuinely devolving appropriate managerial responsibility downwards, at the same time as respecting that some people engaging in campaigns of organisational violence and administrative challenge will require the attention of very senior mangers. The evidence of the respect attributed to the managerial disruptiveness of this group of patients is demonstrated by the management of the 40 or so prisoners in the CSC system being formally overseen by the Home Secretary on a monthly basis, and being operationally managed by a board-level executive.

Staff support and maintenance of team functioning

The third value is the maintenance of team functioning and staff support. Within a group of staff looking after such prisoners, there is inevitably a sequence of individual members of staff being targeted, threatened and vilified, possibly with false accusations, complaints, threats and violence. The creation of an effective team dynamic and functioning will enable a current target to be safely managed in operational practice (for example, by not being on the front line of officers opening a prisoner's cell) and supported by peers both in terms of sympathy as others share experiences of being targeted themselves, and in terms of a group discussion of the possible meaning and motivation of the prisoner group choosing a particular individual. For example, often the person targeted is someone who has been popular and supportive to prisoners, leading to a feeling of jealousy between individual prisoners for that individual. The inter-prisoner rivalry can be resolved by them all turning against the staff member rather than revealing their own sense of vulnerability and dependency. The caustic nature of such psychological violence in tandem with organisationally violent individuals' ability to incite and challenge administrative structures requires genuine teamwork to retain the stability of the staff group functioning.

Rehabilitative focus

The fourth value is the maintenance of a rehabilitative focus. Two underlying values combine to sustain a rehabilitative focus; the first is that people have a right to be managed in the lowest level of security consistent with the level of risk that they present. The second is that the levels of risk that people represent is a pathology that can be mitigated and reduced by therapeutic progress. This might be changes in the attitude of the individual – for example, choosing to cooperate in the development of rehabilitative and managerial strategies for the individual instead of actively attacking and undermining these efforts. The therapeutic progress might be in the effective treatment of underlying mental illness – for example, a reduction in paranoid delusions about the prison officers that has potentiated violence by the individual. This might be in the addressing of risk factors identified from previous adverse incidents – for example, killing in prison – in such a way to reduce that risk and enable return to a less restricted environment. It is possible and probable that individuals will be stuck for long periods in a pattern of hostility and non-engagement in rehabilitative activity, but, even so, the team needs to maintain a clear plan for the individual to get back onto a rehabilitative escalator which the individual can choose to accept or not. Commonly, also, one might expect the individual's degree of engagement to vary, or for further adverse incidents to take place that will trigger a re-evaluation of the presented risk or rehabilitation plans. In such circumstances, it is important as soon as possible for an alternative rehabilitation plan to be developed that takes into account the changed circumstances. It is essential that this is developed as soon as possible, so that the prisoner has a clear sense of choice about how to get out of their destructive spiral and back into making progress.

Respect and openness

The fifth value of respect and openness underpins all the others, and may be the most important attitudinal factor. Maintaining respect towards people who have not respected others by committing crimes is a mark of a civilised society. The management of these difficult individuals demands respect in relation to the potential violence, disruption and damage that they can cause; demands respect to provide a rehabilitative pathway at all times should the individual choose to take it; and demands respect in day-to-day dealings, no matter how much disrespect is thrown back. At a therapeutic level, prisoners in a CSC setting frequently assume that authority is abusive and contemptuous of them, and being fair and respectful without condoning or colluding with their behaviour provides them with a different experience.

Looking at openness, there are three factors involved in this. The first involves openness to the individual about thoughts and discussions about them, and plans for them. From a teamworking perspective it is important to identify decisions as team-based rather than identifying who said what about an individual, so that individuals are not targeted. Within this constraint, openness about plans and thoughts about an individual is important. There is another set of constraints, for example in relation to intelligence received. As far as possible, individuals respond best in full possession of the facts and suspicions about them, so where there are security issues, it would be important to disclose as much as possible as soon as possible. The second involves openness with prisoners' legal representatives. While it is true that there is potential for the development of a toxic mix where a prisoner successfully manipulates a crusading human rights lawyer with a set of half-truths and accusations, it is also true that, firstly, the prisoner's lawyer basically wants the best for their client, as do the CSC treatment team, and, secondly, that if the prisoner is mendaciously instructing their lawyer, this will become clear as the CSC treatment team provide the fuller context of the situation and provide the other side of the half-truths that have been alleged. The natural inclination of staff working with patients in highly restricted environments seems to be to fear enquiry or challenge by their client's legal representatives. The truth of the situation, however, is that prisoners' detention in such circumstances is legitimate, and legal representatives will get a sense of this with a full account of the facts and current situation. Often in these circumstances, the legal representative can become an ally in encouraging the individual to re-engage with the rehabilitative programme that is being offered. It is an interesting but understandable phenomenon that as the lawyer starts to encourage their client to re-engage, that they are sacked. This is probably evidence that the legal challenge was driven more by the motivation of organisational violence or administrative challenge than by a genuine grievance. The third type of openness is to external agencies that have an interest in the practice of the unit, perhaps in terms of human rights, the prevention of torture, racial equality and so on. If a prisoner makes a complaint in relation to one of these issues, then it is important to be open to the scrutiny of the appropriate legitimate investigatory authority, to have confidence that the work being done is not discriminatory or 'cruel and unusual', and that, if there has been a problem, such an external investigation will identify ways in which managers can in good faith improve the service.

Conclusions

In this paper, I have tried to describe something of the culture and practice of the UK Close Supervision Centre system in its efforts to manage the 30 or 40 most difficult prisoners in the UK prison system. I have described the context within which the project was conceived, the developmental states through which it has passed that have evolved practice, and I have discussed the values-based management approach that I believe operates, and which needs to operate when dealing with this exceptionally difficult group of prisoners. The CSC system discharges its duty of care to these most difficult prisoners by working to enable them to de-escalate their dangerous behaviour by exploring its causes; managing them while they are in the grip of it; and all the while creating pathways out of the higher-security setting. I have argued that the potential for such patients to undermine managerial structures should not be underestimated, and that the challenges they present behove the system to be clear about the values on which it is based, and to make itself open to scrutiny of its practice and decisions by prisoners' legal representatives and other interested parties. There is anecdotal evidence that these values and this approach developed in the CSC has informed practice in the management of difficult prisoners elsewhere in the UK prison system, particularly in intensive management (segregation) units. The CSC works in an area where there are not clear models of good practice, nor are there international comparisons of similar services that can be made, and it has been developed largely on the basis of English compromise and pragmatism. I believe that it has itself become a beacon of good practice in this difficult area.

References

Freud S (1936/1966) *The Ego and Mechanisms of Defence.*The Hogarth Press, London.

HM Inspector of Prisons (1999) *Close Supervision Centres. a thematic review.* Home Office, London.

Home Office and Department of Health (1999) *Managing Dangerous People with Severe Personality Disorder: proposals for policy development.* The Home Office, London.

The Prison Rules. Statutory Instrument 1999 No. 728. The Home Office, London.

Department of Health (2000) *The NHS Plan: a plan for investment, a plan for reform.* Department of Health, London.

Wong S and Gordon A (2003) Unpublished draft treatment programme.

Chapter 9

Creating the elements of a humane prison system

Ernest L Cowles

> On Mondays, Wednesdays and Fridays, I walk clockwise around the yard. On Tuesdays, Thursdays and Saturdays, I walk counterclockwise around the yard, like the yin and yang of life, of the universe. I walk whether it's hot or cold, sunny or rain . . . except on Sunday, because the Lord, God Almighty has declared Sunday as a day of rest.
>
> GE, a long-term inmate in a maximum-security prison in the US

Much can be learned about prisons by talking to those who have spent years behind the bars, walls and fences that characterise the fundamental purpose of these institutions. Observations by offenders serving sentences for crimes and those employed to manage and treat the incarcerated provide windows into a place where the observable trappings of the outside community – candy in a visiting room vending machine or a sporting event on the television in a dayroom – belie an alternative world. What becomes obvious through discussions with the keeper and the kept, and observing the physical manifestations of imprisonment is the *totality* of the prison world. Here, *totality* is used to embrace Goffman's (1968) notion of total institutions, but also is meant to convey the notion of *institution* from a larger systems perspective as a close-system organisation that maintains and regulates itself so as to ensure its continuation.

The prison organisation rests on the bed of the society in which it is placed, but it is also clear that prisons are not constructed according to the contemporary images of that society's views of crime, criminals and what should be done about both. Like other social institutions such as the military, education and religious practice, prison institutions are constructed in accordance with current needs, knowledge and technology. Yet, interwoven within these are core values that remain fundamentally static. In everyday experience, the manifestations of popular institutions are often referred to as great traditions, wonderful ceremonies, and remarkable architectural elements. We speak warmly of how these features make us feel secure, give us a sense of pride or connect us with a higher power. When we talk of prisons, however, there is an absence of such positive reflections of core values. Common topics of conversation, even among penal professionals, do not centre on the beautiful gothic architecture of the 'big house', revel in the descriptions of the punishments that have been meted out within the walls of these institutions, or promote the merits of ample prisoner suffering. This is likely because punishment is not a savory topic; yet if we examine prisons, we find remarkable historical consistency in the incorporation of punishment and isolation as core values of the prison as an institution, despite the ebb and flow of public sentiment regarding what should be done with the criminal offender.[1]

Particularly for the better part of the twentieth century, punishment's identity as a core principle of imprisonment has existed primarily as a subtext (see, for example, Johnson, 2002, pp. 60–2). The true nature of prison punishment was fully revealed only when a particularly heinous crime was committed against an innocent, at formal sentencing when a stern judge lectured the convicted about his or her transgressions, or when especially deplorable conditions were discovered in an institution. It was then quickly recast back into an image of humane incarceration, with much fanfare that prison was such an improvement over the past barbaric treatment of offenders, or at least was better than an obliquely referenced 'alternative'. Only in the past couple of decades has the overt recognition of prison as punishment moved to centre stage. Today, it seems punishment is enmeshed in every consideration of prison. Cullen (2001) presents a vivid and chilling assessment of the recent trend:

> [W]e have entered a 'mean season' in which it has become politically correct to build prisons and to devise creative strategies to make offenders suffer. In Todd Clear's words, we are witnessing a movement whose supreme aim is the inflictions of 'penal harm'. (Gillen, 2001, p. 57)

The pre-eminence of 'prison equals punishment' has at least two major implications for a discussion of the future of the institution of prison. First, if punishment is a dominant and enduring core principle of prisons, then the institution of prison will adjust itself to ensure such confinement remains punishing, irrespective of goals such as the provision of treatment. In fact, when goals such as treatment are operationalised in a way that is perceived as antithetical to punishment, formal or informal adjustment mechanisms will reduce or neutralise the conflict. Second, perhaps on a more positive note, the concept that 'prison equals punishment' questions common rhetoric about the programmes that are provided in prison to 'help' the confined unfortunates, and prompts rational discourse about what constitutes 'humane imprisonment'.

The relationship between punishment and treatment

A frequent result of the above noted self-regulation by prisons is a palpable schism between treatment programmes and the security and custody demands of institutions. In Chapter 1 in this volume, Hans Toch ably explores the ramifications of this phenomenon when it comes to implementation of treatment programmes. He points out that effective programmes such as the therapeutic community, which are based in internally established regulation and self-governance, often run into a wall of 'no's when they diverge from the dominant institutional rule structure. My research on the implementation of a juvenile drug treatment therapeutic community (Cowles and Dorman, 2003) affirms and illustrates this, even when the programme is carried out in an institution identified as a treatment facility. The goal incongruities between security and treatment highlighted in that study created the boundaries that isolated the treatment programme and eventually caused its failure. Some of these boundaries were physically manifested:

> Even through the program was located in a juvenile facility, a departmental goal priority on secure confinement was clearly in evidence at the institution. For example, double fences festooned with razor wire typical of today's adult prisons surrounded the institution. Entrance to the institution was gained through a secure sally port, and all employees and visitors were subject to search. Although the facility had an 'open' campus, movement of youth inmates was carefully controlled and under direct supervision. (Cowles and Dorman, 2003, p. 246)

Other boundaries were embedded more subtly in rules, policy and protocols:

> Shortly following program implementation, all program staff was told that DOC security rules were to be enforced and that departmental rules superseded the therapeutic aims. As such, the programme enjoyed little autonomy with respect to security (p. 246).

Situations such as this are not infrequently encountered by researchers and practitioners alike, raising a fundamental question regarding the legitimacy of trying to provide treatment in the prison environment. Fortunately, there is good news in this arena. There is a continuing accumulation of research literature built on meta-analyses indicating the efficacy of treatment (e.g., Andrews, 1995; Andrews, Zinger *et al.* 1990; Dowden and Andrews, 1999a; 1999b; 2000; Garrett, 1985; Izzo and Ross, 1990; Lipsey 1995; Lipsey *et al.*, 2001; McGuire, 2002; McGuire and Priestley, 1995; Wexler *et al.*, 1990; Whitehead and Lab, 1989). The problem is that while the effect size of treatment is statistically significant, it appears quite variable and mediocre. Losel's work (1995) found effect sizes ranging from $r = +.10$ to $r = +.36$ with a mean of about $r = .10$. McGuire (2002) similarly indicates a sizeable variation across treatments with an average reduction in recidivism of 5 per cent to 10 per cent.

A more appropriate answer to the question about the legitimacy of treatment, therefore, seems to be not *whether* we should be undertaking treatment, but *how* we can do it better. I would argue that punishment as currently embedded in the prison system suppresses effective treatment, and systemic changes are needed to reduce its negative impact.

Conditions of effective treatment

Guidance for creating conditions of effective treatment has been emerging from the treatment research. As Dowden and Andrews (2004) emphasises:

> Meta-analytic evidence has suggested the *clinically relevant* and *psychologically informed* [author's emphasis] principles of risk, need and general responsivity are associated with significant reductions in reoffending (p. 203).

Particularly relevant to the discussion here is that the most successful rehabilitation programmes target the risk factors reflecting criminogenic needs. Further, the higher the risk and more intensive the criminogenic need, the more concentrated the treatment regimen needs to be (Dowden and Andrews, 2004). MacKenzie (1999) summarises these core principles into straightforward guidelines for implementation of effective treatment, indicating such programmes should:

- be carefully designed to target the specific characteristics and problems of offenders that can be changed in treatment (dynamic characteristics) and that are predictive of future criminal activities (criminogenic characteristics), such as antisocial attitudes and behaviour, drug use, and anger responses;
- be implemented in a way that is appropriate for the participating offenders and that uses therapeutic techniques known to work (for example, the programme must be delivered as designed, and treatment must be provided by appropriately educated and experienced staff);
- require offenders to spend a reasonable length of time in the programme considering the changes desired (deliver sufficient dosage);
- give the most intensive programmes to offenders who are at the highest risk for recidivism; and
- use cognitive and behavioural treatment methods based on theoretical models such as behaviourism, social learning, or cognitive behavioural theories of change that emphasise positive reinforcement contingencies for pro-social behaviour and are individualised as much as possible.

Unfortunately, in both the US and Great Britain, during the past two decades or so, there has been a forceful movement away from these principles of effectiveness. The promotion of the 'rational choice theory' as a prime component of the larger 'get tough' conservative agenda (see, for example, Burnett and Maruna, 2004) has effectively limited consideration of individualised criminogenic needs by focusing on generalised deterrence and punishment. As a result, the components of effective treatment programming have, in many cases, become hollow. The approach to substance abuse treatment in US prisons provides a good case example of this phenomenon and how it can have a major impact on treatment effectiveness.

The 'get tough on drugs' policy has created an array of mandatory sentences for drug crimes, filling prisons and stretching limited treatment resources far beyond their capacity to remain effective. Over 80% of the increase in the federal prison population from 1985 to 1995 was due to drug convictions (Bureau of Justice Statistics, 1997). Moreover, while the rate of incarceration for drug offences has begun to moderate in the past couple of years, during the two decades from 1980 to 2000 the number of state prisoners incarcerated for drug crimes increased by a staggering 1321 per cent! For comparison, the number of individuals imprisoned for violent crimes increased 339 per cent, and those incarcerated for property crimes rose by 267 per cent, (Beck and Harrison, 2003). Not only did the number of individuals incarcerated for these crimes skyrocket, but the net result seems to have been the catching up of many street-level dealers, who also frequently are users, in a net intended to get drug kingpins. For example, the US Sentencing Commission (1995) indicated that 55 per cent of all federal drug defendants are low-level offenders, such as mules or street dealers, while only 11 per cent are classified as high-level dealers. Essentially, the net result of this massive 'get tough on drugs' campaign has been an overwhelming growth of imprisonment in increasing punitive environments of those involved in drugs at the bottom of the illicit drug food chain. More troubling, the conditions needed for effective treatment of this sizeable proportion of the prison population are simply not being met.

A 1997 survey of the US state prison population found that nearly two-thirds (62.2 per cent) had used drugs, over one in three (36.8 per cent) were using drugs at the time of their offence, and over half (55.1 per cent) were using either alcohol or drugs at the time of their offence (Bureau of Justice Statistics, 1999). The Centre for Alcohol and Substance Abuse (1998) estimates that of the $38 billion spent on corrections in 1996, more than $30 billion was spent incarcerating individuals who had a history of drug and/or alcohol abuse, were convicted of drug and/or alcohol violations, were using drugs and/or alcohol at the time of their crimes, or had committed their crimes to get money to buy drugs. Yet, the majority of this funding is not directed at treatment. According to a US Government Accounting Office report, of the 83 per cent of state prison inmates needing substance abuse treatment, 59 per cent are not receiving any treatment (GAO, 1991). Moreover, the imbalance between treatment need and provision has been growing. In 1997, one in ten State prisoners reported being treated for drug abuse since admission, a decrease from the one in four prisoners reporting such treatment in 1991. There was also a drop in the percentage of Federal prisoners (9 per cent in 1997) reporting treatment since admission (16 per cent in 1991) (Bureau of Justice Statistics, 1999).

More rigorous examination of existing treatment raises additional questions not only of availability but of adequacy. For example, much of what is identified as treatment actually is drug education, which many experts do not consider adequate for the treatment of addiction (see, for example, Lipton *et al.*, 1992). Also, there is a question about 'everything but the kitchen sink' approaches that may serve as facades of treatment with little clinical relevancy (see, for example, Cowles *et al.*,1995, p. 64).

Taken together, these factors support the notion that prison has been over-prescribed as a generic tonic for society's substance abuse problem. Unfortunately this tonic, despite its requisite bad flavour and appearance, has little or no medicinal value as it is currently dispensed. The beneficial compounds, i.e. effective treatment approaches, contained in the tonic have been so diluted in trying to provide them in a mass and imprecise administration that their potency has been lost. Moreover, substance abuse is not the only treatable condition for which generic incarceration seems to have become *de rigueur*. We are seeing, for example, a growing proportion of inmate populations with significant mental health problems who are becoming entangled in the criminal justice system. If prisons are to become humane and effective as change agents, then the principles of effective treatment must be assimilated into their structure. The integration of these principles requires two conditions. First, their assimilation must be externally driven, for without sufficient pressure and support for this change, prisons will remain fixed on what they are now doing well, which is confinement and punishment. Second, this change must be incorporated into the larger prison system, not just individual prison environments. Prisons are well organised into systems to deliver punishment, but are poorly structured to deliver treatment. Programmes such as substance abuse treatment (see, for example, Dowden and Andrews, 2004; Inciardi *et al.*, 1997) require a systematic progression of therapeutic environments matching offender needs. This argues for rethinking where treatment is likely to be most effective: the most secure facilities should have the most intensive treatment programming, for it is within these facilities that those with the most significant criminogenic needs are found.

The growth of increasingly more restrictive and secure prison environments

The previously noted agenda promoting prison time as the dominant means for addressing criminogenic factors such as substance abuse has created 'mandatory minimums' and determinant sentencing structures that have little ability to account for offender change in determining release. Simultaneously, sentencing enhancements, long-term determinant sentences, and habitual offender 'three strikes'-type sentencing structures have combined to keep convicted offenders behind bars for the majority, if not all, of their lives.[2] Due, in large part, to the fact that sentence length is a primary component in determining offender risk in terms of making institutional assignments, the trend of increasing sentence lengths at both low- and high-security ends of the institutional spectrum has led to the 'scaling up' of custody and control functions across the continuum. A noticeable artefact of this scaling up across the institutional continuum is that in the operational world of the prison, the higher the perceived risk, the more controlled and punitive the institution becomes. The following brief vignette offers a personal perspective on this process.

When I was first hired as a young prison psychologist many years ago, I was temporarily assigned to a minimum-security facility for training. The prison previously had been a citrus juice plant and overhead conveyer belts and pipes still connected several of the buildings. Other than the uniformed custody staff, a six-foot high chain link fence with one strand of barbed wire was the only outward sign of its converted purpose. An electric gate which could be fully opened for vehicle traffic onto the compound was left far enough ajar for foot traffic during daylight hours. The only real escapes from the facility were inmates who simply walked out the front gate. By and large, the minimum security environment was designed for individuals who could adjust to an environment where self-control was required.

My recent visits to minimum-security and even youth institutions reveal a very different picture. Double fences with rolls of razor wire strung at their foot and top are commonplace. Electronic surveillance equipment is prevalent, as are 24-hour-a-day floodlights and perimeter patrol vehicles. Often towers manned by armed officers are part of the design. Internal control within these facilities is prominent. Life is well regimented, controlled, and highly structured, and carried out under the constantly watchful supervision of the security staff. In a practical sense, there is very little opportunity or need to exercise self-control or to develop the skills needed for what Robert Johnson has referred to as 'mature coping' (2002, pp. 84–125).

The changes at the high security end of the spectrum are perhaps even more striking. The creation of the 'supermax' prison, as a place where the individuals in need of the highest security and most supervision are confined, stands as testimony to the abject notion of efficient and secure imprisonment. Originally, such units were constructed as wings or small units within existing maximum-security institutions designed to hold a few of the most problematic of the inmates within that facility. Today, more and more of these supermax units are being developed to hold a wide variety of problematic inmates, not only from within a larger institution, but also as a destination for inmates across a larger prison system. A study published by the National Institute of Corrections in 1999 (Riveland, 1999), found more than 30 states were operating a supermax facility or were planning to open one. The supermax prison is a place where life has been reduced to the barest essentials. It is perhaps best revealed not by what is seen, but by what is not seen, in these facilities. Although there is considerable variation in operations and programming across the US in these facilities (Riveland, 1999), they share characteristics of austere environment and omnipresent, some might say invasive, security. There is little movement or interaction. Most confine individuals to cells 20 to 23 hours a day, and most feed residents within their cells. Officers monitor the inmates' movements by video cameras. When prisoners are permitted out of their cells for a brief hour of exercise or a shower (usually three times a week or less) they are handcuffed, shackled and escorted by two or three correctional officers. Communication between prisoners and control booth officers occurs mostly through speakers and microphones. For the confined, privacy is in short supply. One-piece sinks/toilets are located in a corner of the cell, visible from the door window. Nothing is permitted in the cells that would, in any way, obstruct the officer's view of the prisoner in the cell or that could possibly be used to fashion a weapon. Even non-threatening personal effects such as pictures are tightly regulated for 'security' purposes. The offender has almost no control of his/her environment. Commonly, an officer at a control centre may be able to monitor cells and corridors and control all doors electronically. Lights are controlled by officers outside the cell, and often are left on 24 hours a day. Contact with the outside world has been reduced to carefully selected and controlled opportunities. There are no contact visits (prisoners sit behind a Plexiglas window) and phone calls and visitation privileges are strictly allocated. Books and magazines may be denied. TV and radios, if allowed, can only receive certain channels, and staff can typically remotely control them. Although the units are frequently air-conditioned, it is because many have no windows and windows, if present, are fixed shut.

In the present day, this 'supermax' prison has replaced the 'cat o' nine tails' and the 'hole'. Puréed, but nutritiously acceptable, food has replaced the bread and water diet. Five-point restraints have replaced leg irons and wall manacles. Yet today, prisons from low-security to maximum-security have created environments of what I will call *benign deprivation*. To understand benign deprivation and its genesis, it is necessary to consider the bureaucracy of the prison system. Like all bureaucracies, prisons and prison systems are reactive: they respond to and defend themselves against both internal and external threats. On one hand, if secure confinement is an overarching goal of prisons, then today's technology makes it possible to achieve that goal with some assurance. Internal threats to custody and control have been countered by technology, which has been used to ratchet up the barriers between the convicted and the community and to control these individuals inside prisons. Essentially, the pains of imprisonment (Sykes, 1958) have become interwoven into the fabric of the prison through this technology. On the other hand, the courts have become an increasingly major external threat to the prison bureaucracy. During the past 40 years or so, the courts have taken an activist approach to remedying the ills of prison conditions. Since the reversal of earlier federal and state 'hands off' policy toward prison conditions in the 1970s, judicial activism has resulted in court control of major prisons in nearly every state in the US at some time, with eight states having their entire prison systems under court control (Morris, 1995, p. 245). Such loss of control is anathema to the bureaucratic institution of prisons. Indeed, as James Jacobs indicates, one of the likely impacts of prisoner rights litigation has been the increased bureaucratisation of the prison:

> Until recently, prisons operated as traditional, nonbureaucratic institutions. There were no written rules and regulations, and daily operating procedures were passed down from one generation to the next. Wardens spoke of prison administration as an 'art'; they operated by intuition . . . Early lawsuits revealed the inability of prison officials to justify or even to explain their procedures. The courts increasingly demanded rational decision-making processes and written rules and regulations . . . The prisons required more support staff to meet the increasing demand for 'documentation'. New bureaucratic offices and practices began to appear.
>
> (Jacobs, 2001, p. 222)

In a somewhat ironic twist, the same technology which has entrenched deprivation as a means of achieving elevated security and control also has provided the prison bureaucracy the means to skilfully adjust the conditions of confinement to meet court-mandated requirements vis-à-vis the Eighth Amendment threshold against 'cruel and unusual punishment'. However, once a legal mandate has been neutralised, the prison bureaucracy returns to its state of equilibrium or rest; for once the required remedy has been attained, there is little bureaucratic interest or need to improve conditions beyond court-identified minimums.

It is the nexus of these two countervailing forces, court oversight and the maintenance of a secure, punitive environment that has created the conditions for benign deprivation. Bureaucratic expediency requires that prisons provide the mandated essentials, yet the same pragmatism directs that anything that does not ultimately contribute to prisons' real mission of custody be stripped away. Stated differently, intentional cruelty largely has been replaced by organisational expediency.

The need for clear distinctions between conditions of confinement and treatment

Possibly because of the lack of effective treatment conditions and the benign deprivation discussed above, the distinctions between conditions of confinement and treatment have become increasingly murky. This is particularly true in two instances. The first involves identifying the basic services provided in prisons as treatment. More and more often, functions associated with the basic health and wellbeing of inmates are being promoted as treatment. To understand this trend, it is first necessary to consider the concept of treatment. As conceptualised here, the basic question is whether the programme or services labelled 'treatment' attends to an identified criminogenic problem. For example, while medical care could conceivably deal with an underlying pathology associated with criminal behaviour, e.g. the removal of a tumour causing aggressive behaviour or medication to assist in easing of withdrawal symptoms, the majority of medical services provided in prison are directed toward the same fundamental health issues faced by individuals in the free world. In fact, the primary reason that medical services are made available in prison is because confinement precludes inmates from securing medical care through other venues. Nonetheless, as Welch (2005) notes, some 'penal harm' proponents maintain medical care is a luxury and prisons should limit their commitment to healthcare to take full advantage of the punitive nature of imprisonment. While this position may represent the extreme, it reflects the problem which occurs when the basics of humane incarceration, such as medical care, are considered benefits rather than essentials. From this point, it is a simple leap of logic to classify almost any activity or service provided for inmates as therapeutic. Thus, merely providing a humane environment is presented as curative, and being in prison itself is viewed as the necessary and sufficient condition to bring about offender change.

The second instance comes when prison officials restore that which was artificially deprived. I am not referring to the practice of removing privileges for disciplinary infractions, then permitting the individual to regain those privileges through demonstrated positive behaviour. Behaviourist psychology has demonstrated that a well designed series of contingencies can effectively shape behaviour – providing the punishment is not arbitrarily inflicted, that clear associations exist between the infliction of the punishment and the undesirable behaviour, and that clear associations exist between positive behaviour and its rewards. Rather, I am referring here to the situation of artificially depriving the incarcerated individual of basic comforts, then allowing the prisoners to earn back those essentials. Such programmes, often popular in the 1960s and 1970s, were frequently presented as a form of behaviour modification called the 'token economy'. While many of these programmes had legitimate systems of rewards, frequently the programmes started by artificially depriving the individual of basic services and programmes that would have been provided had he or she not been a participant. This included depriving individuals of 'privileges' such as daily showers, visitors, and reading materials. In more severe cases, deprivations included blankets, clothing, toothbrushes, and sleep. By the mid 1970s, such practices and even more extensive problems with other forms of behaviour modification, including the use of aversive therapy and electroshock therapy, brought national attention to the abuses perpetrated under the guise of this therapeutic approach. The Prison Project of the American Civil Liberties Union challenged an experimental programme known as START (Special Treatment and Rehabilitation Training) located at the US Bureau of Prisons in Springfield, Missouri (Neier, 1974), and in 1975 a major national symposium was held on the topic (McCrea, 1975). Because of these combined efforts and additional lawsuits, the harsher and more severely corrupted of these approaches were eliminated. However, recent incarnations of such programmes have again begun to appear in the form of 'earned privileges' programmes at prison boot camps and in supermax facilities. Without sound theoretical underpinnings, such programmes merely become ways to justify depriving the imprisoned of fundamentally humane conditions.

Making time in prison meaningful

During this discussion, I have deliberately tried to avoid the use of the term 'correctional institution' in place of 'prison' for two reasons. First, I believe it blatantly misrepresents the current nature of prisons. Second, it subtly reinforces the image that prisons can become increasingly punitive without being harmful and can simultaneously treat all offenders effectively. Such representations lead away from true substantive discussion of the primary goal of incarceration, the relationship between punishment and treatment, the quality of life in prison and other legitimate issues concerning the future of the prison institution. How then can we proceed without getting tangled in emotionally laden rhetoric that accompanies the concepts described in this chapter? I suggest that one approach to consider is the question: can we make time in prison meaningful?

The question of meaningful time immediately shifts the focus of imprisonment away from the crime and onto the offender. It further puts a context around the discussion of both punishment and treatment and puts boundaries on each. Moreover, the notion of meaningful time does not support conditions of imprisonment that undermine effective treatment. Perhaps most importantly, it requires an honest examination of the value of the prison sentence. Life in today's prison world is filled with unproductive time for not only the inmate but the staff as well. Few, even among the most ardent supporters of severe punishment, would agree that this unproductive time has value. It creates 'penal harm' and wastes resources. Perhaps because unproductive time is so prevalent among those serving major portions of their lives in prison, it is easier to see the problem in this sub-population of inmates. These offenders typically come into the prison environment and then go through an intensive programming phase. They frequently engage in a gamut of available programmes – counselling, basic or secondary education, perhaps even college, life skills offerings, vocational training – only to find that after successfully completing these, they are still an inmate, still imprisoned and still facing a multitude of years in behind bars, walls, and fences. Beyond a prison job, however, there is little to productively occupy their time. Most, such as the individual cited at the beginning of this discussion try to impose meaning in their lives by developing routines to consume time. These routines take on a ritualistic significance to the individual, but ultimately speak to the futility of life without purpose.

We must strive to build prison systems that can make prison time meaningful if we are ever to achieve humane imprisonment. To do so will require changes that prison systems are themselves incapable of addressing, because they cannot change without external support to redefine their primary purpose away from punishment. For shorter-term inmates, this means convincing the community that development of effective treatment environments and programmes is more in its interest than simply having the offender pay for the crime. For longer-term inmates it requires rethinking how secure prisons can provide productive lives for the worst of humanity.

References

Andrews DA (1995) The psychology of criminal conduct and effective treatment. In: J McGuire (ed) *What Works: reducing reoffending – guidelines from research and practice*. Wiley, Chichester.

Andrews DA, Zinger I, Hoge RD *et al.* (1990) Does correctional treatment work? A clinically relevant and psychologically informed meta-analysis. *Criminology*. **28**: 369–404.

Beck A and Harrison D (2003) *Correctional Populations in the United States, 1997, and Prisoners in 2002*. Bureau of Justice Statistics, US Department of Justice. US Department of Justice, Washington, DC. www.ojp.usdoj.gov/bjs/glance/tables/corrtyptab.htm.

Bureau of Justice Statistics (1999) *Substance Abuse and Treatment, State and Federal Prisoners, 1997*. US Department of Justice, Washington, DC.

Bureau of Justice Statistics (1997) *Correctional Population in the United States, 1997*. US Department of Justice, Washington, DC. www.ojp.usdoj.gov/bjs/pub/pdf/satsfp97.pdf.

Burnett R and Maruna S (2004) So 'prison works', does it? The criminal careers of 130 men released from prison under home secretary, Michael Howard. *The Howard Journal*. **43**(4): 390–404.

Centre for Alcohol and Substance Abuse (1998) *Behind Bars: substance abuse and America's prison population*. Columbia University, New York, NY.

Cowles EL and Dorman L (2003) Problems in creating boundaryless treatment regimens in secure correctional environment: private sector-public agency infrastructure compatibility. *Prison Journal*. **83**(3): 235–57.

Cowles EL, Castellano TC and Gransky LA (1995) *'Boot Camp' Drug Treatment and Aftercare Intervention: an evaluation review*. US Department of Justice, National Institute of Justice, Washington, DC.

Cullen FT (2001) Assessing the penal harm movement. In: E Latessa, A Holsinger, JW Marquart and JR Sorensen (eds) *Correctional Contexts: Contemporary and Classical Readings* (2e). Roxbury Publishing, Los Angeles, CA.

Dowden C and Andrews DA (2004) The importance of staff practice in delivering effective correctional treatment: A meta-analytic review of core correctional practice. *International Journal of Offender Therapy and Comparative Criminology*. **48**(2): 203–14.

Dowden C and Andrews DA (2000) Effective correctional treatment and violent reoffending: a meta-analysis. *Canadian Journal of Criminology.* **42**: 449–76.

Dowden C and Andrews DA (1999a) What works for female offenders: a meta-analytic review. *Crime and Delinquency.* **45**: 438–52.

Dowden C and Andrews DA (1999b) What works in young offender treatment: a meta-analysis. *Forum on Corrections Research.* **11**(2): 21–4.

Garrett CJ (1985) Effects of residential treatment of adjudicated delinquents: a meta-analysis. *Journal of Research in Crime and Delinquency.* **22**: 287–308.

Goffman E (1968) *Asylums: essays on the social situation of mental patients and other inmates.* Penguin, Harmondsworth. (First published 1961, Doubleday Anchor, New York, NY.)

Inciardi JA, Martin SS, Butzin CA *et al.* (1997) An effective model of prison-based treatment for drug-involved offenders. *Journal of Drug Issues.* **Spring**. Available at: www.udel.edu/butzin/articles/effect.html.

Izzo RL and Ross RR (1990) A meta-analysis of rehabilitation programmes for juvenile delinquents: a brief report. *Criminal Justice and Behaviour.* **17**: 134–42.

Jacobs JB (2001) The prisoners' rights movement and its impacts. In: E Latessa, A Holsinger, JW Marquart and JR Sorensen (eds) *Correctional Contexts: Contemporary and Classical Readings* (2e). Roxbury Publishing, Los Angeles, CA.

Johnson R (2002) *Hard Time: understanding and reforming the prison* (3e). Wadsworth, Belmont, CA.

Lipsey MW (1995) What do we learn from 400 research studies on the effectiveness of treatment with juvenile delinquents? In J McGuire (ed) *What Works: reducing reoffending: guidelines from research and practice.* Wiley, Chichester.

Lipsey MW, Chapman GL and Landenberger NA (2001) Cognitive behavioural programmes for offenders. *Annals of the American Academy of Political and Social Science.* **578**: 144–57.

Lipton DS, Falkin GP and Wexler HK (1992) Correctional drug abuse in the United States: an overview. In: C Leukefled and F Tims (eds) *Drug Abuse Treatment in Prisons and Jails.* National Institute on Drug Abuse, Research Monograph No. 118. US Department of Health and Human Services, National Institute on Drug Abuse, Rockville, MD.

Losel F (1995) The efficacy of correctional treatment: A review and synthesis of meta-evaluations. In: J McGuire (ed) *What Works: reducing reoffending: guidelines from research and practice.* Wiley, Chichester, UK.

Maurer M, King RS and Young MC (2004) The meaning of 'life'. Long prison sentences in context. The Sentencing Project, Washington DC. www.sentencingproject.or/pdfs/lifers.pdf.

McCrea R (1975) *Modification and its Discontents: the national conference on behavioural issues in closed institutions.* The Capital Times and Alicia Patterson Foundation, Madison, WI.

MacKenzie DL (1999) Commentary: the effectiveness of aftercare programmes – examining the evidence. *Juvenile Justice Bulletin: Reintegration, Supervised Release, and Intensive Aftercare.* US Department of Justice, Office of Juvenile Justice and Delinquency Prevention, Washington, DC.

McGuire J (2002) Integrating findings from research reviews. In: J McGuire (ed) *Offender Rehabilitation and Treatment: effective programmes and policies to reduce re-offending.* Wiley, Chichester.

McGuire J and Priestly P (1995) Reviewing what works: past, present and future. In: J McGuire (ed) *What Works: reducing re-offending – guidelines from research and practice.* Wiley, Chichester, England.

Morris N (1995) The contemporary prison. In: N Morris and DJ Rothman (eds) *The

Oxford History of the Prison: the practice of punishment in Western society. Oxford University Press, New York, NY.

Neier A (1974) A programme to cripple federal prisoners. *The New York Review of Books.* **21**(3). www.nybooks.com/articles/9589.

Riveland C (1999) *Supermax Prisons: overview and general considerations, National Institute of Corrections, US Department of Justice.* US Department of Justice, Washington, DC.

Sykes GM (1958) *The Society of Captives: a study of a maximum security prison.* Princeton University Press, Princeton, NJ.

US General Accounting Office (1991) *Drug Treatment: state prisons face challenges in providing services, Report to the Committee on Government Operations, House of Representatives.* US Congress, Washington, DC.

US Sentencing Commission (1995) *Special Report to Congress: cocaine and federal sentencing policy.* US Sentencing Commission, Washington, DC.

Welch M (2005) *Ironies of Imprisonment.* Sage, Thousand Oaks, CA.

Wexler HK, Falkin GP and Lipton DS (1990) Outcome evaluation of a prison therapeutic community for substance abuse treatment. *Criminal Justice and Behaviour.* **17**: 71–92.

Whitehead JT and Lab SP (1989) A meta-analysis of juvenile correctional treatment. *Journal of Research in Crime and Delinquency.* **26**: 276–95.

Notes

1 For an excellent review see, Morris N and Rothman DJ (eds) (1995) *The Oxford History of the Prison: The Practice of Punishment in Western Society.* Oxford University Press, New York, NY.

2 According to the Sentencing Project (Maurer *et al.*, 2004) in the US: one of every 11 offenders in state/federal prison (9.4 per cent or 127 677 persons) is now serving a life sentence; of the lifers in prison, one in four (26.3 per cent) is serving a sentence of life without parole, having increased from one in six (17.8 per cent) in 1992; the number of lifers in prison rose by 83 per cent from 69 845 in 1992 to 127 677 in 2003; and time to be served for lifers admitted to prison increased by 37 per cent between 1991 and 1997, rising from 21.2 years to 29 years.

Chapter 10

Women's imprisonment: how getting better is getting worse

Sunny Marriner and Dawn Moore

> I hate your jails, I hate your bars
> I hate your chains, I hate this law
> That got women in the shadows, sisters behind the shade
>
> Faith Nolan, 2001

Incarcerated women are oft described as 'too few to count', a depiction which holds true for the entire western world. Women, as Nolan points out, live in the shadows of the criminal justice system. This shadowing means that incarcerated women have been subject to enduring discrimination, alienation, abuse and neglect. When women prisoners are noticed (as with the establishment of women-only prisons in the nineteenth century) their treatment has oscillated between victimising, patronising, marginalising, and stereotyping.

Canadian punishment has recently attempted to extract itself from the long-established practice of shadowing imprisoned women. Coming off a rocky century of human rights abuses in women's prisons, in the late 1990s the Canadian Government ushered in sweeping changes to the practice of punishing women in this country. The punishment of women in Canada today is informed by a rhetoric of *choice* and *empowerment* and is said to be guided by feminist principles and visions of creating 'woman-centeredness' in the penal system. Indeed, the punishment of women (and more recently girls) in Canada is often positioned as a sort of global benchmark, as woman-centeredness is proselytised across Europe and North America. The new age of punishing women in Canada is not without its critics, however. Many decry the new model as veiling its own forms of cruelty, marginalisation, and discrimination (see, for example, Hannah-Moffat, 2001; Hannah-Moffat and Shaw, 2000; Monture-Angus, 2000). The Correctional Service of Canada (CSC) was recently the target of a successful human rights complaint citing racism and sexism in the so-called woman-centered practices. Feminist activists and academics who were integral to the process of change in the early 1990s are calling foul, citing co-optation of their ideals and a bastardisation of the original vision.

The intention of reformers in the 1990s was doubtless to do better by women incarcerated in Canada. The concern is that the bid to do better, while alleviating some of the key concerns about women's imprisonment, also brought new concerns to the fore. Particularly worrying is the use of risk/need assessment schemes, enduring problems with security classifications, and psychological/rehabilitative interventions. We start with a brief overview of the history of women's punishment in Canada in order to set the stage to introduce and outline the changes brought about in the mid-1990s. We then move to concerns emerging out of these changes. As part of the expansion of the woman-centered initiative, girls in conflict with the law in Canada are the newest additions to the practice of 'empowering punishment'. (The feminist notion of empowerment [or helping people to access their own agency] was injected into the Canadian women's penal schema in the late 1980s. We discuss this in more detail below.) Drawing on our first-hand experiences and observations working within custodial environments, we then focus the lens more closely on some of the effects of the woman-centered model on the lived reality of girls and young women in conflict with the law.

Imprisoning women in Canada

For 70-odd years the Prison for Women (P4W) in Kingston, Ontario was the main prison for federally sentenced women in the country.[1] The prison's dubious history (well documented by Hannah-Moffat, 2001) endured to its closure in 2000 . Throughout the 1980s, concerns about the conditions in P4W increased. Self-injury and suicide were increasingly common (six Aboriginal women killed themselves in a two-year period). As the only prison for federally sentenced women in the country, P4W housed women whose families and children lived thousands of miles away, making contact almost impossible. There were few employment and training opportunities and those that existed were gendered (e.g. offering hairstyling as vocational training). The conditions at P4W prompted a federal task force investigation. In their April 1990 report, *Creating Choices*, the Task Force on Federally Sentenced Women (TFFSW, 1990) recommended the closure of P4W and the erection of five new regional women's facilities. In addition, they called for a shift in penal practice concerning women, noting that women's experience of imprisonment was qualitatively different than that of men and thus women ought not be subjected to the male model.

The report was more or less shelved until P4W came under public scrutiny in 1996 as the result of a widely publicised and criticised strip search and cell extraction of six female prisoners by an all-male riot squad. In the aftermath a Royal Commission (Arbour, 1996), headed by then Madam Justice Louise Arbour, spent a year reviewing the events at P4W and the experience of federally incarcerated women in Canada generally. In her final report, Arbour sharply condemns what she calls the 'culture of lawlessness' that pervades Canada's prisons and called for sweeping change to the Service including the establishment of a 'culture of rights.'

The events at P4W coupled with Arbour's scathing report served as a catalyst to hurry along the changes outlined by the TFFSW. Today, the P4W is closed and five regional women's facilities stand in its place. The new prisons claim woman-centeredness as their guiding principle, an idea that informs location, architecture, management, and programming. The notion of woman-centeredness originates in the feminist critiques of the penal system that argued that prisons were imagined, constructed, and operated based on a male norm. That is, the prison as an institution was built by men, to service men. Alongside the fact that prisons were neither imagined nor designed to house women, there is strong evidence to support the suggestion that women experience imprisonment differently than men and that women prisoners constitute a population with different needs (Kendall, 1994; Martel, 2000). Women's prisons have yet to imagine adequate responses to pregnancy or women's roles as primary (and often sole) caregivers. Women in prison have astoundingly high rates of history of trauma and abuse. The most widely cited figure from the Canadian Association of Elizabeth Fry Societies (CAEFs, 2001) suggested that 82% of all women and 90% of Aboriginal women in prison have experienced sexual or physical violence. More women in prison self-injure than men, an action often initially developed as a response to abuse, trauma, and isolation, and now extended as a means of coping with the similar powerlessness of prison life.

In answer to these critiques, the five regional women's facilities were opened in the late 1990s, spread across the country so as to lessen the degree of geographic isolation. The prisons are built on the cottage model, housing women in townhouse-like structures as opposed to ranges (the Canadian version of a cell block). The prisons intended to offer lower levels of security and greater freedom of movement within the prison grounds as well as a dynamic and individualised response to criminality. Responding to the lack of access to Aboriginal cultural traditions, one new facility was designed in the model of an Aboriginal Healing Lodge. In keeping with CSC's model of effective rehabilitative initiatives, core criminogenic programming based on the Cognitive Behavioural (CBT) tradition is implemented at all these facilities. Women are streamed into these programmes through an elaborate, actuarial risk/need assessment. These sweeping changes were imagined to create prisons that would empower women rather than subjugate or abuse them and teach them how to make good, 'pro-social' choices in their lives.

The reality of these prisons has been quite different.

Assessment

Following the scheme for male prisoners devised by CSC in the early 1990s, all federally sentenced women undergo a lengthy assessment process that evaluates the woman prisoner's levels of security and recidivism risk as well as identifying what are termed 'criminogenic needs,' or rehabilitative target areas. The assessment is largely actuarial and meant to respond to concerns about sex discrimination by offering a gender-specific, objective measurement of risk and need. However, critical analysis of the assessment process reveals that it is neither objective nor free of discrimination.

Hannah-Moffat (1999) argues that the police reports, pre-sentence reports, criminal records, and reasons for sentencing included in the risk assessment are hardly objective sources. On the contrary, these reports are products of subjective, legal processes that have themselves tended to discriminate against women who fail to meet the imagined norm of a white, middle class, well behaved, maternal woman. Case management officers are also given ultimate veto power over the risk/need assessment scheme, meaning that the final decision is subject to what CSC calls 'professional discretion.'

This subjectivity, as Hannah-Moffat observes, serves to reinscribe age-old stereotypes about what makes a 'good woman.' Married women, educated women and women with histories of stable employment are all 'lower risk' under this scheme.

What is most concerning about the risk assessment schemes is that they are wedded to the assessment of a woman's 'needs.' The mandate of responding to women's needs is born out of the lack of response characteristic of the history of women's prisons. While we applaud the intention to offer a holistic response to the considerable needs of women prisoners (educational, trauma recovery, spiritual, cultural, and so on), needs, under the rubric of CSC, however, have become risks. The assessment process is meant to establish a risk/need profile of a woman whereby her needs and risks correlate, such that one designated high need is, by definition, high risk. We challenge any best practice that suggests that a woman ought to be held at a higher level of security or denied parole because, for example, she disclosed to her case manager that she was sexually abused as a child, grew up poor and may now use substances as a form of self-medication.

Security

Equally concerning are the effects of the risk assessment schemes on women's security ratings. A prisoner's security rating in the federal system is arguably the single most important factor in determining her quality of life while incarcerated. The security rating determines institutional placement (i.e. maximum, medium or minimum), form of housing (i.e. dorm, cottage, range or segregation) and the prisoner's 'privileges' while incarcerated (i.e. freedom of movement, frequency of access to visitors, institutional job placement). We learned nothing from the hard-taught lessons of P4W if we fail to appreciate that the practice of holding women in high security is all too easy and all too destructive. At P4W most women were held in conditions far more secure than necessary (and there is certainly an argument to be made that all women were held in conditions that far exceeded the threats they posed). The effect was disastrous as women engaged in self-mutilation and suicide attempts (many of which were successful) in order to escape from the oppressive conditions.

The so-called objective risk assessment scheme introduced by CSC was meant, among other things, to address the overclassification of women as high risk. The aftermath of its implementation suggests that this is not in fact the case. In 2004, the Canadian Association of Elizabeth Fry Societies (CAEFS), as part of a coalition of groups concerned with women's equality, launched a human rights complaint against CSC and the Canadian Government. The complaint cites both racist and sexist discrimination within the practice of incarcerating women. One of the most enduring and acute areas of concern is the incarceration of Aboriginal women.

Fifty per cent of federally incarcerated Aboriginal women are classified as maximum security compared with 8–10 per cent of their non-Aboriginal counterparts, illustrating that patterns of discrimination in the security rating process persist. In the CAEFS submission Monture-Angus explains the origins and effects of the overclassification of Aboriginal women as high risk. Here (Monture-Angus, 1999) she pays particular attention to the assessment of 'community functioning.'

Too often, the norm is that Aboriginal people do not belong to communities that are functional and healthy, thanks to colonisation. Therefore, constructing a 'community functioning' category ensures that Aboriginal people will not have access to scoring well in this category. This is not a factor for which individuals can be held solely accountable. Rather than measuring risk, this dimension actually merely affirms that Aboriginal people have been negatively affected by colonialism. What is being measured is not 'risk,' but rather one's experience as part of an oppressed group.

While these concerns are raised about Aboriginal women we want to be clear that they speak to broader ethnocentricities that affect all culturally marginalised women. Pollock (2000) raises similar worries about the effects of cultural insensitivities on incarcerated women of colour. Because the risk assessment tools are not culturally specific, they fail to appreciate the many and varied forms of community building, support and positive growth found in culturally marginalised communities. For example, shared parenting (where a community shares the responsibility of childrearing) is often reframed through western eyes as child neglect.

Security concerns have further reinscribed the 'too few to count' mentality for those few women labelled high security risk. Because the regional facilities are designed to house low- to medium-security women, the women deemed in need of high security are still housed in men's institutions, a practice clearly condemned in both the TFFSW report (1990) and the Arbour Commission (Arbour, 1996). These few women suffer the same fate as those imprisoned at P4W (and indeed some are the same women), wherein they have few programming options, are isolated and held in oppressive conditions. The results here are equally concerning as these women manifest the same troubling and self-harming behaviours that characterised P4W. The fact that Aboriginal women and women of colour are more likely to be classified as high-risk further amplifies these worries. The CSC is aware of the problem but has yet to come up with an adequate solution, and continues to use the men's prisons as a stopgap measure (even as the gap is ever-expanding).

Programming

The ultimate purpose of security rating and risk/need classification within the penal model pioneered by CSC is the administration of 'targeted criminogenic programming' aimed at reducing a woman's risk of recidivism. The standardised programme model for women is organised around two central principles of woman-centeredness: empowerment and the creation of meaningful and responsible choices. The effect of implementing system-wide programmatic changes has been to create what Moore and Hannah-Moffat (2004) term a 'liberal veil' whereby appearances of woman-centeredness and cultural specificity are well maintained but practices reveal a decidedly less progressive approach.

Our primary concern is the apparent paradox presented in conjuring an initiative meant to forcibly confine and restrict while simultaneously establishing an environment that empowers women to make independent choices about their lives. The prison setting, by its very definition, is one that negates choice. Prisoners are told when to wake, eat, bathe; whom they might visit; what services they can access; where they will live; when they will leave; which traumas are worthy of attention and how they should heal from those traumas. The 'meaningful choices' left for women in prison are sparse. The choice between disclosing one's childhood sexual abuse or being denied parole, for example, is hardly empowering or meaningful.

Programmes are meant to teach prisoners 'coping skills' to assist them in reintegration and the establishment of a 'non-criminal' lifestyle when they are returned to the community. The reality, however, is that prison life is vastly different from community life, troubling the transfer of these 'skills'. The skills taught in prison are meant to facilitate a 'pro-social' lifestyle among women. This is based on the assumption that women's criminality is inherently antisocial and somehow irrational. Women's own understanding of their crimes give a notably different account. Pollock (2000) in her study of women of colour in prison illustrates this point. One woman explains that she would rather steal to feed her children than go and ask for money from a man. As Pollock points out, the behaviours exhibited by this woman are positive, pro-social and independent. She desires to care for her children and wants to be able to provide for them on her own. The choice to steal rather than be kept is a strong, independent, rational choice.

The gap between the liberal rhetoric of empowerment and free choice that has become the hallmark of CSC's vision of punishing women, and the reality of women's experiences of imprisonment is palpable. On paper it appears that CSC has embraced feminist principles in shaping programming. On the ground, however, it is clear that feminist argot has merely been co-opted. Empowerment and meaningful choice are recruited as tools of lip service that serve to obscure the continuation of the same practices they are meant to remedy (Hannah-Moffat, 2000; Shaw, 1999). Not only do practices that further disempower federally sentenced women become obscured by the veneer of progress, but these same practices are now trickling into other penal spheres. In recent years penal schemes aimed at young women and girls have come to increasingly resemble these same initiatives with the same worrying results.

Too few to count, and still fewer?

If adult women are 'too few to count' within a larger correctional body, then custodial realities in the detention and custody of teen women act as an extreme illustration of the distorted actualisation of the 'woman-centered' model. Females make up less than 15 per cent of youth in custody and fewer than one in five youths in detention or on probation (http://canada.justice. gc.ca/en/ps/rs/rep/1998/tr98-4a.html – 25 July 2005). Ribboned throughout the system of incarceration for teen women are all the themes that have come to characterise the punishment of adult women. Primary among these is the championing of 'treatment' models as representing a kinder, gentler correctional system. The use of the word 'treatment' to describe everything from behavioural modification to involuntary drugging effectively creates a smokescreen behind which many historic prison abuses have re-emerged. Prevailing rehabilitative theory, however, provides an air of legitimacy, and even 'best practices', to techniques that are questionable at best and, many argue, abusive at worst.

The pathologisation of women's responses to trauma

The review of the shifts in perspective, as they relate to punitiveness versus treatment, demonstrates the correctional move away from seeing criminality in the context of environment and social factors. The current practice of identifying 'criminogenic needs', as the foundation of reducing recidivism and criminal behaviour generally, illustrates an overall societal trend – similarly evident in correctional culture – of the pathologising of the individual. As such, treatment practices converge around the theory that individual 'thinking errors' or irrationality cause antisocial behaviours and 'pro-criminal senti-ment' and thus a correction in *individual thinking* is desired. While this approach is heralded as an advance in understanding rehabilitative factors, it simultaneously represents a devaluation of decades of accumulated feminist theoretical and practical work establishing the links between women's experience of violence and their subsequent criminalisation. Kendall (2000, p. 82) makes the point clearly:

> Specifically, my attempts to acknowledge structural problems such as racism, sexism, classism, and violence were ultimately transformed into pathologies lying within individual women prisoners . . .

The CBT/criminogenic need approach to assessing criminality is disturbing, in that it separates a woman's context of abuse and violence from her subsequent 'needs' and life circumstances. When a range of 82–90% of incarcerated women and girls report experiencing physical or sexual violence(www. elizabethfry.ca/eweek00/factsheet.htm – 26 July 2005) one must necessarily question the 'woman-centeredness' of any approach that treats this informa-tion as incidental. Further, very real dangers emerge when notions of 'treat-ment' are introduced in settings that are explicitly based on power and control, the fundamental roots of violence against women. This broadly opens the door for revictimisation and retraumatisation through the very tools designed to 'correct' what are viewed as cognitive errors, but are instead normative responses to trauma or, in the language of the front-line women in this field, reasonable responses to unreasonable circumstances.

By orienting specific responses to trauma as maladaptive cognitive misfires we see a shift in thinking back to much-challenged victim-blaming theories that prevailed in early psychiatric interventions with childhood sexual abuse survivors. Rather than recognise the prevalence of abuse, particularly sexual abuse, of women and children as a societal problem that we as communities have a responsibility to address, we instead focus on demanding the survivor change *her response* to violence. This, in effect, allows us to shirk our collective responsibility for addressing abuse against women and children, viewing it instead as a *static factor*: that which exists as an element of risk, but is deemed unchangeable and thus not relevant as part of 'treatment.' This phenomenon can be summed up quite aptly by one incarcerated survivor's challenge to the institution's 'treatment' of her perceived 'anger-management needs':

> If I hit you in the head over and over and over again, and then you turn around and hit me back, does the problem get fixed if I make you write a 'thinking report?'

Youth, and young women in particular, are notably vulnerable to the hazards of the thinking-error theory of criminality. Societal attitudes about the rights of the individual are moderated in the case of youth, in that the adult populace perceives itself as bearing a responsibility and entitlement to 'correct' and 'reshape.' In light of this, popular opinion embraces far greater latitude in the treatments, practices and medical interventions considered appropriate for the state to impose upon youth. In custodial settings, this perception of entitlement has acquired a veil of nurturance and child protection. As such, intrusive interventions, rights deficits cloaked in the rhetoric of 'safety,' and chemical experimentation all enjoy a defended space in youth penality.

For the young detained or sentenced woman, this conceptualisation of incarceration as treatment is still more fraught with risks when taken in conjunction with gender specificity. The reframing of coping strategies and reactions to abuse as 'mental health needs' or 'disorders' is notably higher with young women; and thus the tendency to employ chemical and diagnostic approaches is elevated. Young criminalised women's responses to abuse make them more likely to be diagnosed with depressive, anxiety/panic, and obsessive-compulsive disorders than their male counterparts; and their socialised responses of expressing trauma through means such as self-injury and body-image/eating issues are exacerbated by the power and control functions of custody. As a result, studies of incarcerated young women in the US advance the notion that fully three-quarters of detained girls have psychiatric disorders, as contrasted with an estimated 15% of the general (mixed) youth population (www.nimh.nih.gov/Press/prjuveniles.cfm – 25 July 2005).

The tendency to view women's response to trauma as evidence that psychological fragility is inherently tied to gender is a long-established sexual stereotype found within the 'helping' and medical professions (Breggin, 1991; Burstow, 1992; 2005; Caplan, 1985). Generations of abused women seeking support through therapy, psychology, and psychiatry report the unwelcome experience of having their reactions repositioned as disorders and their coping reframed to support notions of women's greater emotional instability (Burstow, 1992; Caplan, 1995; 2005). In a closed custodial setting, reasonable responses for female survivors of sexual or physical abuse are regularly transformed into evidence of security risk or 'mental health issues.' As survivor-based responses tend to be routinely triggered by experiences of powerlessness, perceived threat, and enforced silencing of means of expression, the prison environment itself is often inherently emotionally unsafe or retraumatising for a majority of girls and women within it. Kendall (2000, p. 82), in her study of the experiences of women in prison, concludes that:

prisoners identified the pains of imprisonment to be not only contrary to therapy and rehabilitation but also the greatest contributing factor to their emotional distress.

The day-to-day operational environment of custody, with its regular manifestations of loss of physical and emotional agency, may lead to near-daily triggered responses for female survivors of violence.

Treaters or keepers?

The culture of treatment can further lend itself to an alarmingly blurred role for custodial staff. The conception of 'treatment' as the inverse of 'punishment' has created a framework in which the keepers can perceive themselves as 'helpers,' and thus reinvent power and control structures as beneficial to the sentenced young woman. With an emphasis on programming and CBT advocated as the role of the custodial 'youth worker,' young incarcerated women are increasingly pressured to disclose sensitive and vulnerable information to the same individuals who hold the keys that control their movements. Thus the keeper with whom a young woman may be asked to discuss her experience of childhood sexual abuse is also the person who locks her in her room or strip searches her later that day. All power and control over her physical needs such as eating, sleeping, bathroom and personal hygiene access, and even menstruation,[2] is in their hands. This level of physical control combined with heightened, and oft-times involuntary, emotional vulnerability can obfuscate the boundaries between safe and unsafe exposure in a manner that may be eerily reminiscent of the originating abuse. When we acknowledge that violence against women and girls is rooted in an attempt to gain and maintain power, it is conclusive that support or therapy around it cannot replicate the very conditions it seeks to address.

A further concern with this blurring of the lines arises when keepers believe it to be their role to 'correct' young women, particularly in the area of comportment, sexual attitudes, and value systems. The notion that particular behaviours, outside of criminal activity, are preferable for young women carries with it the broad risk of imposing oppressive gender roles that hark back to early prison models. Conventional female morality that dictates 'appropriate behaviour' for girls, *as envisioned by the keepers*, still underscores many of the messages young incarcerated women receive in day-to-day programming and institutional life. For example, a young woman who has multiple sexual partners may no longer be told she is promiscuous *per se*, but she may regularly hear messages that tie 'having respect for herself' to the number, gender, and 'quality' of people she chooses to be intimate with. Not only does this advance a specific view of women's sexuality and their choice to exercise it, but it further implies a notion of societal agreement on the role and comportment of women which is, in reality, anything but consensus-based. To institutional staff, however, an implied responsibility to create healthy, pro-social girls might also mean a duty to reorganise value systems that, in reality, have nothing to do with criminality. The inclusion of a category referencing sexual behaviours on most youth risk assessment tools merely lends support to the notion that keepers are expected to probe non-criminal, subjective factors when 'supporting' a young woman through the system. These problems of role confusion are on the upswing with increased provincial movement to privatised youth facilities, and a lack of meaningful provincial legislation mandating the presence of distinct clinical staff in youth custodial environments.

The security catch-all

As discussed above, individual security classifications raise the problem of distinct inequities for sentenced women and girls (see CAEFFS, 2001; 2003). Concerns about incarcerated girls must also include careful consideration of the lack of uniform definitions for youth facility classification. While publicly available Correctional Service of Canada policy documents offer a startlingly general description of what factors constitute minimum-, medium-, and maximum-security federal institutions, there appears to be an even greater deficit in specific uniform definitions for provincial youth facilities. The common terminology used to refer to levels of custody for youth diverges from the level-based minimum, medium, and maximum; and instead tends to employ only 'open' and 'secure-custody' as primary descriptors. This more generalised language results in a difficulty determining what specific living conditions and levels of restriction are considered appropriate for sentenced youth. Compounding the vagaries in determining uniform standards for security classification is the fact that youth correctional services in Canada are administered differently in different provinces, with variance in risk assessment tools, private versus publicly operated facilities, and how young offenders are housed (Hannah-Moffat and Maurutto, 2003). Consequently, in some regions detained and sentenced youth are held together, young women and men are held in coed facilities, and what might be deemed 'minimum-' and 'maximum-' security prisoners are in the same units under the same restrictive conditions. Despite the lack of transparency around 'security' and what it is intended to mean in relation to young offenders, security is the most regularly cited rationale behind day-to-day operating procedures, privileges, and restrictions under which they live. Even in cases where conditions appear to have been made less restrictive for youth, compensatory security measures may negate any benefit they might have enjoyed. For example, provincially incarcerated young women who are permitted daily full contact visits with family members may then be subject to mandatory strip-searching following each visit. As a result young women are placed in a position of deciding between contact with loved ones and maintaining their integrity of person. For those who have histories of sexual assault or abuse, the cost of the degradation of forced inspection may simply be too high and thus compel them to regularly forego visitation while in custody. Had they been held in a less 'permissive' facility, they would have access to secure visitation, meaning no subsequent strip search would be required. Thus we see how the elements often lauded as hallmarks of a 'kinder, gentler' system may create untenable choices that have the practical effect of increased punitiveness for young women.

A further illustration of the security conundrum extends to young women's ability to express themselves within the custodial environment. In adult correctional environments there are strict policies regarding Institutional Crisis Intervention Teams (ICIT) and cell extraction teams. Indeed, some of the most egregious rights violations of federally sentenced women first came to light through their use, as highlighted by the Arbour Commission (Arbour, 1996). In contrast, youth correctional institutions (particularly those that are privately run by transfer payment recipients) are subject to different policies and correctional oversight and thus ICIT and other emergency teams may be entirely absent. The differences in these formalised responses are often touted as evidence that we are treating youth less punitively and under less threat, and thus subjecting them to gentler conditions. The day-to-day operational reality of this may, however, be the inverse. The lowered access to on-site crisis response is instead used to justify greater, not less, restriction of basic freedoms for youth. For example, in many facilities all conversations between young women are closely monitored under the auspices of security, and they are immediately penalised, and sometimes segregated, if they speak outside the hearing of institutional staff. Thus, when walking in line from one part of the institution to another, or when staff are at a distance in living units, young women are required to maintain silence. If two young women share an ethnic background and speak a first language other than English or French, they may be forbidden to converse with one another in their language of fluency and must instead speak in the language of the staff present. This restriction edges past repression and borders onto the discriminatory when the elevated custodial numbers of racialised girls who speak English as a second language are considered.

Additionally, the content of conversations between young women is often closely restricted. In many youth facilities young women are not allowed to discuss: their crime or sentence; where they live; information about parents or siblings; who their friends are; who they may be dating; or indeed, nearly any information about their lives on the outside. Rationales for this range from protecting them from themselves (in that young offender identities are protected under Canadian legislation), discouraging pro-criminal thoughts and sentiments while in custody, and preventing association with one another post-release. The practical reality is that young women, who tend to rate relationships to friends and family as a highest value, may be virtually forbidden to acknowledge their most important connections, even when those are considered 'pro-social' by assessment standards. This not only stifles their ability to communicate about what is meaningful to them, it exacerbates the experience of isolation, loss of identity, and disconnection from community – an effect that directly contradicts the desired goals of most international perspectives on juvenile justice.

Concerns around security may further be used to limit access to writing implements and private journals. Young women are often granted access to written expression only between scheduled daytime hours, and not during times of high agitation or distress when they are arguably most necessary. Night-time is highlighted as a particularly vulnerable time for abuse survivors, and particularly those incarcerated. Support models for survivors often use journaling as both a positive form of self-expression, and a grounding mechanism when women are experiencing nightmares, flashbacks, thoughts of self-injury, etc. The justification for the restriction on writing implements has again been linked back to lowered access to ICIT and cell extraction teams – the presumption being that young women allowed to keep pencils in their cells overnight might use them to attack institutional staff, or injure themselves. When the security card is played in this way it is not uncommon for keepers to relanguage it as 'a safety issue,' implying that it is somehow for the young women's own good. Ironically, in our private interactions with incarcerated young women, they regularly link their own aggressive, self-injurious or suicidal responses to the effect of being forced to internalisze traumatic responses. They point to the silencing effected by restricted verbal expression, access to writing, and the reading of their journals for 'security reasons,' as causal factors in heightened stress, emotional 'outbursts,' and conflict with staff and other inmates. While most facilities imposing such restrictions claim they are non-intrusive and respectful of privacy, it is our own observation that young women have lost privileges and even been penalised through segregation for 'inappropriate' thoughts, expressions of anger, or drawings in journals. Not only does this enforce that anything ranging outside the label deemed 'pro-social' must be kept carefully hidden and unexpressed while in the custodial environment, it further sends young women the distinct message that nothing, not even your thoughts, is allowed to be private. Should they deviate, even in thinking and regardless of behaviour, from institutional compliance, they may be consequenced and further stigmatised by everyone from institutional staff to probation officers who may oversee them in the community for years to come. The implication is that external compliance and non-criminal behaviour can never be enough. Instead, prevailing correctional practice not only claims the right to imprison young women, it further demands that they agree with their imprisonment. To be fully considered 'pro-social,' a young woman must not only be seen to support her own subjugation, ideally she would even be thankful for it.

Conclusion

When examining the practical outcomes of an idealised vision for women's corrections, we see that laudatory goals of woman-centeredness do not equate to better imprisonment. The moving and personal testimonials of so many federally sentenced women, so explicitly offered to the TFFSW and the Arbour Commission, in the end could not be translated into meaningful and supportive practice when filtered through correctional culture. What were deemed woman-centered approaches have instead cloaked old concepts in new language, without altering systemic failings in a framework never meant to reflect women's ways of being and learning. Treatment has become punitive when married to structures of control, lower-security environments have merely widened the net over who is classified 'high-risk,' and choices have become requirements in order to be considered compliant and, ultimately, allowed to go free. Many times over in the last 15 years, equality-seeking groups have celebrated reports, commissions, and policy reviews from myriad levels of government that claim to acknowledge discrimination against women under Canadian correctional practice, and promise sweeping change. Most recently in 2004, the Canadian Human Rights Commission completed a systemic review of human rights violations of women prisoners, as a result of a complaint filed on behalf of federally sentenced women (discussed above). The resultant report, 'Protecting Their Rights: A Systemic Review of Human Rights in Correctional Services for Federally Sentenced Women' (CHRC, 2004) contained 19 recommendations for change that once again reinforced and elaborated on the findings in Arbour and *Creating Choices*. In response, the Correctional Service of Canada released an Action Plan in February 2005 that was embraced and endorsed by CHRC but broadly criticised by the original complainants as falling far short of a real commitment to address the abuses. The complainants further expressed their distress that the CHRC appeared to have no real intent to require CSC to comply (www.elizabeth-fry.ca/submissn/csc-humr/1.htm – 7 March 2005). In July 2005 the Office of the Correctional Investigator released a preliminary analysis of CSC's Action Plan, finding that most changes and recommendations are not implemented or are implemented imperfectly, that timelines have been extended many years in the future, and emphasising in particular that women-centered expertise is once again missing (www.oci-bec.gc.ca/reports/Response_CSCAP_e.asp – 18 July 2005). Thus we see that the repetitive cycle of analysis, study, and recommendation is moving women in Canada no further ahead, and instead asks them to do the same work again and again, in the guise of consultation. Again and again we find the resulting picture of women's imprisonment looks the same as ever it did. This reality insists that at this point it can only be considered futile to continue adding new recommendations or reiterating old ones. All of the evidence reflects that new iterations of old problems will not be the axis point for change in women's criminality. Instead, the collected voice of Canadian women seems to demand the question of whether imprisonment can ever be an effective means of responding to women's crimes or if it is time to embark on a new vision, without bars.

References

Arbour L (1996) *Commission of Inquiry into Certain Events at the Prison for Women in Kingston (Arbour Report)*. Public Works and Government Services of Canada, Ottawa.

CAEFS (2001) *The Risky Business Of Risk Assessment*. www.elizabethfry.ca/risky/Contents.htm.

CAEFS (2003) Submissions to the Human Rights Commission. Special report on the discrimination on the basis of sex, race and disability faced by federally sentenced women.

Caplan PJ (1985) *The Myth Of Women's Masochism*. New American Library, New York.

Caplan PJ (1995) *They Say You're Crazy*. Perseus, Reading.

Caplan PJ (2005) Sex bias in psychiatric diagnosis and the court. In: W Chan, DE Chunn and R Menzies (eds) *Women, Madness and the Law*. GlassHouse Press, London.

CHRC (2004) Canadian Association of Elizabeth Fry Societies. Submissions to the Canadian Human Rights Commission by Representatives of National Equality-Seeking Groups Regarding the Systemic Review of Human Rights. Violations of Women Prisoners by the Government of Canada. CD ROM.

Breggin PR (1991) *Toxic Psychiatry*. St. Martins Press, New York.

Burstow B (1992) *Radical Feminist Therapy: working in the context of violence*. Sage, Newbury Park.

Burstow B (2005) Feminist antipsychiatric praxis: women and the movement(s): a Canadian perspective. In: W Chan, DE Chunn and R Menzies (eds) *Women, Madness and the Law*. GlassHouse Press, London.

Hannah-Moffat K (1999) Moral agent or acturial subject? Risk and Canadian women's imprisonment. *Theoretical Criminology*. **3**(1): 74-91.

Hannah-Moffat K (2000) Prisons that empower: neoliberal governance in Canadian Women's Prison. In: *British Journal of Criminology*. Winter: 510–31.

Hannah-Moffat K (2001) *Punishment in Disguise: penal governance and federal imprisonment of women in Canada*. University of Toronto Press, Toronto.

Hannah-Moffat K and Mauretto P (2003) *Youth Risk/Need Assessment: an overview of issues and practices.* Department of Sociology, UTM, University of Toronto. http://canada.justice.gc.ca/en/ps/rs/rep/2003/rr03yj-4rryj-4.html

Hannah-Moffat K and Shaw M (eds) (2000) *An Ideal Prison? Critical essays on women's imprisonment in Canada*. Fernwood, Halifax.

Kendall K (1994) Creating real choices: a programme evaluation of therapeutic services at the Prison for Women. *Forum on Corrections Research*. **6**(1): 19–21.

Kendall K (2000) Psy-ence fiction: governing female prisons through the psychological sciences. In: K Hannah-Moffat and Shaw (eds) *An Ideal Prison? Critical essays on women's imprisonment in Canada*. Fernwood, Halifax.

Martel J (2000) Women in the hole: the unquestioned practice of segregation. In: K Hannah-Moffat and Shaw (eds) *An Ideal Prison? Critical essays on women's imprisonment in Canada*. Fernwood, Halifax.

Moore D and Hannah-Moffat K (2004) The liberal veil: revisiting Canadian penality. In: Pratt *et al.* (eds) *The New Punitiveness: trends, theories, perspectives*. Willan, London.

Monture-Angus P (1999) *Women and Risk: aboriginal women, colonialism and correctional practice – some preliminary comments*. Workshop on Gender, Diversity and Classification in Federally Sentenced Women's Facilities. Toronto.

Monture-Angus P (2000) Aboriginal women and correctional practice: reflections on the Task Force on Federally Sentenced Women. In: K Hannah-Moffat and Shaw (eds) *An Ideal Prison? Critical essays on women's imprisonment in Canada*. Fernwood, Halifax.

Nolan Faith (2001). *Live with Mary Watkin*. (Album)

Pollock S (2000) Dependency discourse as social control. In: K Hannah-Moffat and Shaw (eds) *An Ideal Prison? Critical essays on women's imprisonment in Canada*. Fernwood, Halifax.

Shaw M (1999) Knowledge without acknowledgement: violent women, the prison and the cottage. In: *Howard Journal of Criminal Justice*. **38**(3): 252–66.

Task Force on Federally Sentenced Women (TFFSW) (1990) *Creating Choices*. Solicitor General, Ottawa.

Notes

1 In Canada, penal responsibilities are divided between the federal and provincial governments. Those serving custodial sentences exceeding two years come under federal jurisdiction. Youth, probationers and anyone serving two years less a day come under provincial responsibility.

2 In many custodial settings young women have to request access to feminine hygiene products and the number of requests they make are logged and communicated across shifts.

Chapter 11

Governing a humane prison

Peter Bennett

Introduction

Just before I arrived at Grendon in September 2002, I recall receiving congratulatory letters from two of my predecessors who between them had notched up 17 years of governing the prison. 'Welcome to the best governing job in the world,' wrote one. It felt as if I had been granted an exceptional privilege: the responsibility of safeguarding a unique tradition in a very special kind of prison.

I soon became aware of another, more distant, presence. I learned that the imposing portrait of an eighteenth century naval captain which hung above my desk was the penal reformer, Captain James Maconochie, a man whose 'extraordinary vision', according to a recent biographer, 'saved transported convicts from degradation and despair' (Clay, 2001). In the 1840s Captain Maconochie governed a notorious penal settlement on Norfolk Island, 1000 miles east of New South Wales, accommodating 'the absolute worst of the system'. He introduced reforms in the treatment of prisoners which have since been commended for being ahead of their time. Unfortunately, Maconochie's experiment was short-lived and he was recalled, his good work surviving as an inspiration if not a reality. The portrait had hung for many years in the governor's office at Grendon, presumably as an example for the compassionate treatment of prisoners and yet simultaneously a solemn reminder of the vulnerability of experimental penal reforms.

It is often said that governors set the moral tone of the prisons they manage (see, for example, Narey, in Liebling, 2004, p. 398). Like naval captains they carry a heavy responsibility, exercising considerable moral leadership within the confines of a remote world where the potential for the abuse of authority is ever-present. Indeed, the governor's influence should never be underestimated. Person and role are not easily disentangled. Humanity can be captured in bureaucratic standards and prison rules, but it also resides, and must be seen to reside, in the hearts of those who exercise power over prisoners.

But it is also the case that governors find the wherewithal to manage humanely, or otherwise, in the people, institutions and cultures over which they have control. Some prisons, it appears, are more humane than others. I have managed a prison where I was regularly beset with obstacles to regime reform in favour of a perceived need by a powerful faction among staff to establish strict order and control. In another prison I had the more satisfying task of developing an experimental regime for managing difficult and disruptive prisoners, allowing them a significant degree of choice in their participation (Bennett, 1991). Sadly, the Hull Special Unit has shared the fate of many penal experiments, although, like Barlinnie, it provided valuable lessons for the recent development of special and DSPD units at Woodhill, Whitemoor and Frankland. Captain Maconochie's legacy is testimony to the fact that experiments are seldom completely wasted, reforms accumulate incrementally, albeit invariably there are difficulties in prolonging them in practice.

I am therefore particularly fortunate as I write to be the current governor of a prison which has shown an extraordinary resilience over the 43 years of its existence, and this despite real and perceived threats from outside as well as destructive tendencies from within. Grendon, a therapeutic community prison in Buckinghamshire, England, has received wide acclaim for its staff–prisoner relationships and, as I am always fond of repeating to visitors, kept alight the flame of rehabilitation during the dark decades of the 1970s and 1980s. Lord Justice Woolf described the disturbances at Strangeways, Manchester, and in many other prisons in 1990, as a reaction to impoverished regimes and inhumane, unjust treatment of prisoners (Woolf, 1991). Grendon typically provided a refuge from this storm.

But Grendon, being a prison in which incidents are rare, is not necessarily any easier to manage. Slick, top-down managerial efficiency is often considered by staff and prisoners to be damaging to a regime which places a high value on consultation, openness and democratic decision-making processes. Grendon is a particularly complex and difficult prison to manage, mainly because of the cultural and structural tensions arising from the uneasy coexistence of democratic, and would-be autonomous, therapeutic communities within an hierarchical, encapsulating Prison Service. Grendon is a highly specialised kind of prison which is nevertheless managed by a mainstream governor who is required to support the therapeutic process while yet ensuring its conformity with the rest of the Prison Service. The two forms of organisation could not be more dissimilar. The achievement of a healthy and lasting *modus vivendi* is a continuing challenge.

I intend to show that Grendon is, by any standards, a humane prison whose expressions of humanity are determined by, and embedded in, the therapy. Humanity is preserved in the fabric of the therapeutic tradition. A governor appointed to manage this tradition needs to demonstrate acute sensitivity to its workings if he/she is to protect the therapeutic programmes and their moral accompaniments from clumsy interventions from outside and self-destructive tendencies from within. The governor must manage between, on the one hand, the expectations of the Prison Service, often expressed in the language of managerialism and, on the other hand, the principles of group psychotherapy, articulated in an adapted vocabulary of equality, democracy and autonomy. This chapter is therefore about my role as governor in understanding, managing, nurturing, protecting, developing, adapting and brokering a penal tradition which embodies a highly distinctive form of humane containment.

Grendon Therapeutic Community Prison

Grendon opened in 1962 as a 'unique experiment in the psychological treatment of offenders' (Genders and Player, 1995, p. 5), including those with mental disorders responsive to treatment as well as of those diagnosed as psychopaths. Particularly distinctive was that during the first two decades Grendon existed on the periphery of the Prison Service, being managed by a medical superintendent. However, following a review by an advisory committee (ACTRAG) set up by the Home Secretary in 1984, Grendon's purpose was defined more clearly with reference to the treatment of 'sociopaths', sex offenders and long-term/lifer prisoners, and the medical superintendent was superseded by a traditional Prison Service governor grade with a senior medical officer as Director of Therapy reporting to the governor. The appointment of a Prison Service governor heralded a critical change to the therapeutic tradition which has continued to have repercussions until the present day. Genders and Player regret the erosion of medical authority in the face of a 'managerial revolution' in the Prison Service (1995, p. 227). This chapter allows me an opportunity to provide another take on this continuing tension.

At present Grendon remains a category B prison for adult male offenders who volunteer to engage in therapy for a period of at least two years. There are five therapeutic communities of between 40 and 46 prisoners and an assessment unit which holds up to 25 prisoners. The regime is centred on community meetings and small group work with complementary programmes of psychodrama and art therapy. The approach is essentially multidisciplinary. Prisoners are expected to engage in group therapy over a prolonged period. Groups are organised on democratic lines and considerable autonomy is invested in communities.

Grendon as a humane prison

To describe a prison as humane can be highly subjective. Senior Prison Service managers often say how they can feel the atmosphere and mood of a prison as if by a sixth sense. I do not intend to spend time here defining humanity in a penal context. Ideas of what is humane can be culture- and time-specific. Moreover, humanity becomes apparent from the ways it is expressed. Various institutions, cultures and patterns of relationships define and express what is humane, or what approximates to our idea of humane, in different ways. Similarly, humanity, as well as the experience of humanity, can thrive in a range of penal organisations; in Grendon humanity is inextricably tied up with, and embedded in, the therapeutic tradition. The therapeutic structure shapes the distinctive moral climate and culture of the prison.

I should explain further. For example, the present Director General and his predecessor would have no difficulty in accepting Woolf's idea of a humane prison. Indeed, they have both taken great pains to promote values of decency and respect in the way prison staff treat prisoners. Decency and respect are built into key performance targets, standards and the auditing process. Indeed, the recent development of the Measuring the Quality of Prison Life survey (MQPL) or measuring the moral performance of prisons (see Liebling, 2004) 'has taken us beyond the measurement of quantity, beyond the measurement of quality of process into the measurement of the quality of relationships, which lies at the moral heart of imprisonment' (Wheatley, 2005, p. 34). Prisoners are surveyed on, among other things, dimensions of respect, humanity, relationships, trust, fairness, order, security and safety. Moreover, it goes without saying that the justification underlying the humane treatment of prisoners is that humane containment and positive regimes lead to successful resettlement and lower reconviction rates which means less crime and greater reassurance of public protection. In Grendon, all of the above prevails as part and parcel of government policy and Prison Service practice. But humanity is also, and has long been, intrinsic to the principles and expected behaviours of the therapeutic regime. Equality of treatment, democratic decision-making, respect for personal autonomy, mutual support, individual welfare, protection and care for the individual who has suffered by way of past traumatic experiences are all ideals specifically developed within a distinctive psychodynamic therapeutic process. The construct of humanity as defined and practised by the Prison Service nationally and humanity as it emerges from therapy at Grendon belong to two overlapping, albeit very different, spheres of discourse, the one which presumes to be universal and which is clearly political, rational and utilitarian, the other which is a mix of the medical, the therapeutic and the psychoanalytical, which presumes to be distinctive and which nevertheless can lead to the same rehabilitative outcome. Indeed, many would consider the therapeutic programme at Grendon to be a more successful way to rehabilitation, for beyond the alleviation of individual suffering through group therapy comes greater self-understanding, self-esteem and self-control and hence greater likelihood of resettlement and ultimately more effective public protection. In short, at Grendon there has been traditionally a greater emphasis on treatment of the individual with public protection as an inevitable and significant by-product. Some staff and prisoners would argue that the focus on the individual is being overtaken by a political agenda which emphasises resettlement, reconviction rates and risk assessments. This inevitably invites the riposte: what about humanity for the victims, the public? And so the debate goes on with 'humanity' being located in different contexts and redefined accordingly.

Given the embeddedness of humane treatment in the therapeutic tradition at Grendon, I have become acutely aware that changes to the structure within which therapy operates could influence the moral climate in which staff and prisoners act out therapy for good or ill. It also follows that the idea of sharing good practice, of exporting bits and pieces of the Grendon tradition to other prisons, is more easily said than done, since transported seedlings of humanity are unlikely to take root unless they have similar therapeutic structures in which to germinate. This is what I mean by humane treatment being embedded in the therapeutic tradition.

And this is why Grendon has been widely acclaimed as a humane prison. A recent report by the Chief Inspector of Prisons was highly positive in this respect, describing Grendon as being an 'exceptionally safe' prison, where staff 'rarely had to resort to use of force' and 'the therapeutic process had led to exceptionally good staff–prisoner relationships' and all this in a prison in which 'a high proportion of men [are] popularly known as psychopaths'. Aware of the tensions inherent between a therapeutic prison and the wider Prison Service, the report endorsed recent attempts by management to balance therapy with security, the need to ensure order and control (HMCIoP, 2004).

Similarly, a recent Measuring the Quality of Prison Life survey conducted by the Prison Service Standards Audit Unit had some remarkable findings which compare very favourably with surveys conducted in other prisons (HM Prison Service, 2004). For example, 91 per cent of prisoners agreed that 'they felt they were treated with respect by staff in the prison' (2 per cent disagreed); 91 per cent agreed that 'most staff treated them with kindness' and 79 per cent that 'they were treated as a person of value in the prison'; 72 per cent disagreed that 'some of the treatment they received in the prison was degrading'; 91 per cent agreed that 'relationships between staff and prisoners . . .was good'. In conclusion, the report acknowledged prisoners' 'extremely positive' comments about the therapeutic community regime, expressing confidence that the prison is doing all it can to prevent prisoners' re-offending and that 'staff were friendly and showed a genuine concern for their well-being'. Besides some criticisms, such as the poor wages and lack of gym facilities, it is significant that prisoners 'felt the security of the prison was too rigid', even though it is manifestly the case that physical security at Grendon is relatively unsophisticated (HMCIoP, 2004, p. 4) and that security procedures are particularly unobtrusive when compared with other category B prisons. Some prisoners' comments reflect a view at Grendon that security, backed up by the operational line of the Prison Service, the governor and the Security Department, often serves to constrict therapy in a context where trust and responsibility have greater efficacy.

The MQPL survey, despite its positive findings, could be criticised for reinforcing the Prison Service's, and by extension the government's, alleged preoccupation with measurement. Perhaps this is one of the most recent expressions of what Genders and Player regard as managerialism, with its potentially erosive qualities. But I believe that, as a Prison Service governor, given the task of achieving performance targets as well as delivering therapy, it is pragmatic to demonstrate as forcibly as possible how well Grendon is achieving in a wider comparative context. After all, measured success is acknowledged success is credible success. It is a safeguard for the present and the future.

I welcomed the MQPL survey of Grendon, having been disappointed by a narrow statistical approach to measuring success in terms of reconviction rates alone. This is why I sponsored a seminar in December 2004, 'Measuring Grendon', which focused on a wide variety of ways that Grendon could be judged as being a successful prison. I pointed to the low incidence of self-harm and bullying, the absence of serious incidents, the scarcity of hard drugs, the very occasional resort to use of force as a means of control, the absence of a segregation unit and the positive nature of prisoner–staff relationships. Grendon, having striven in the past to distinguish itself from the wider Prison Service, has been rather too reticent to engage in wider penal debate and has therefore missed out on valuable opportunities to promote itself and its strategic significance at a national level. It is therefore particularly important that Grendon now asserts itself in the emerging world of the National Offender Management System because it has a great deal to offer in the treatment of prisoners with personality disorders hitherto often dismissed as being untreatable.

Organisational dynamics

In my recent experience, governing a humane prison is about governing a therapeutic community prison since humanity is articulated by, and part of, the Grendon therapeutic tradition. Moreover, I argue that attempts to understand the dynamics of the encapsulating and the encapsulated in terms of the Prison Service and therapeutic community structures are helpful in explaining tensions generated, as well as pointing towards how such tensions might be addressed by a manager tasked with the protection, preservation and promotion of the therapeutic tradition.

My understanding of the role of governor within this highly complex milieu is bound to be subjective to some degree. After all, I am hardly likely to recommend the removal of the governor and the reappointment of a medical superintendent as a reasonable way forward. Although prison governors form a broad church, I am sure the Director General is comforted by their overall commitment to mainstream policies and practices.

I do believe, however, that my background as a social anthropologist provides me with the conceptual wherewithal to enhance my understanding of the governor's contextual role at Grendon. While I cannot presume to keep the objectivity of a field researcher, I feel confident that I have a degree of self-awareness that enables me to locate my position among the socio-cultural forces at work at Grendon as well as to show a respect for the diverse views expressed, and positions adopted, by my significant role-others. Thinking role-free is my own form of transcendentalism; I become an actor embroiled in the thick description of my own ethnography. It is also comforting and stressbusting for, thinking in this way, my frustrations are better managed, placed in a context which renders the actions of others more meaningful.

Given this anthropological perception, I have found it helpful and relevant to compare the therapeutic communities at Grendon with a form of social grouping which has received considerable attention in the literature – the sect. I have noted elsewhere that sects have become central to some highly influential thinking on social process (Bennett, 1993, pp. 3–7). Weber invented the concept of 'charisma' and its 'routinization' and distinguished analytically between 'sect' and 'church' types (Weber, 1947, pp. 358ff.). Focusing on Reformation Christianity, Troeltsch identified a dialectical process involving the world-compromising tendencies of the church and the world-rejecting tendencies of the sect (Troeltsch, 1950). Noting the absence of an established church in America, Niebuhr (1929), introduced the concept of 'denomination' and 'denominationalism' as the process by which sects undergo reconciliation with the world. Sects rarely retain their radical identities beyond the first generation. Voluntary adherence diminishes as members become more likely to accept the standards and morality of the wider society. Highly distinctive, experimental, set-apart and charismatic at the outset, sects gradually seek a position of compromise and accommodation within the dominant society. Members mourn the loss of charisma but realise that in order to preserve the original charismatic experience it must become embedded in bureaucratic rules, procedures and liturgies. Paradoxically, the sect adopts the bureaucratic structures which it once rejected in order to preserve its pristine experiences, albeit such experiences are transformed, routinised.

I refer back continually to my experiences of sectarian dynamics when participating in the daily dramas as they are acted out in Grendon, particularly in the various meetings from wing to senior management level. The resemblance of sect to therapeutic community, of the church or denomination to the Prison Service, as well as the dialectical relationship between them is particularly revealing. Take, for example the following table of characteristics:

Table 11.1

Therapeutic community/sect	Prison Service/established church
• democratic/egalitarian (communitarian/ congregational) • exclusive • autonomous/world rejecting • nonconformist tendencies • multidisciplinary/fellowship of saints • charismatic cult figures • voluntary membership	• bureaucratic/hierarchical • inclusive • accommodating/world-compromising • conformist, adherence to rules of established order • bureaucratic stratification/ritual hierarchy • bureaucratic administrators/ritual intermediaries • non-voluntary membership, i.e. by sentencing and allocation or by birth

Thus, we have the sect which is typically egalitarian, often recruiting members from among the socially deprived and oppressed, encouraging the removal of priestly hierarchies and valuing the participation of all in a tight-knit community of the faithful, whose members are voluntary initiates who reject the morality of the outside world, as well as the authority of priestly intermediaries in response to the transcendent call of the gospel, and who demonstrate a spontaneity of devotion which sets them apart as special. In comparison, we have the therapeutic community, which aspires to be 'democratic' in its decision-making, albeit 'threatened by the overarching penal context' (Genders and Player, 1995, p. 222), which recruits many of its members from prisoners who are socially rejected and regarded as untreatable, disruptive or difficult; which encourages the participation of staff and prisoners in intimate group and community meetings; whose members are volunteers, who tend to denigrate the Prison Service as the 'System', being purportedly inhumane and ineffective as a means of rehabilitation and who express distrust of senior Prison Service officials whom they accuse of trying to 'make Grendon a System prison'; and who practise an openness and spontaneity of personal expression within the small groups which helps them to change their lives forever.

The above table represents extremes, each grouping demonstrating, to a greater or lesser degree, the tendencies listed. I do not wish to labour the resemblances; I believe I have made a point. Suffice it to mention that many members of a sect and members of a therapeutic community share one very special thing in common: an intensely emotional personal and life-changing experience amounting to 'conversion'.

Synchronically, then, the therapeutic community prison, like the sect, sits uncomfortably within the encapsulating social order, continually debating when to make compromises and when to oppose external interference. During my time, such debates have centred on attempts to introduce drug counsellors, proposals to set up a cognitive skills course for sex offenders to run alongside the therapeutic regime, enhancements to the regime by introducing accredited work programmes during the afternoons, the implementation of more comprehensive security procedures and the introduction of a new baton to be worn by uniformed staff. As each issue arises, so differences of opinion emerge.

Diachronically, the evolution of the therapeutic community over time reflects an inevitable and gradual process of routinisation as Grendon has been expected to conform with the increasing managerial initiatives of the Service, with their reliance on audits, standards and performance targets. This process also informs what amounts to a distinctive perception of time articulated by Grendonites in terms of a continuing external threat to restrict, or to destroy altogether, the therapeutic tradition. Typically, this is presented as a view of better past times, a Golden Age, which has been, and is being, inevitably compromised and eroded. In Therapy Forum, a weekly meeting open to all staff, degeneration is often voiced in terms of a sense of irrevocable loss accompanied by despair and inevitably raising within me, as governor, a variety of emotions, ranging from guilt and hurt to frustration and defiance.

And so factions emerge, fade and re-emerge; new alignments form as issues change. But perspectives often coalesce around particular groupings. Prisoners understandably will bemoan the loss of the privileges which a therapeutic security prison bestows. Therapists will fight to preserve Grendon's core psychodynamic principles. Threats from within may be typically located in new staff, particularly if there is a significant influx of prison officers who have not had time to assimilate the tradition, or with new managers tutored and trained in performance management. Even psychologists, who have an active and intimate involvement in group therapy, may be seen as posing a threat if they show an unhealthy reliance on cognitive principles and risk assessments. And foremost of all those who might wreak havoc is the governor, the interloper who superseded the medical superintendent.

The role of governor, then, is one of understanding such organisational variances, of respecting the views, misgivings and fears of staff and prisoners, and of striving to achieve a compatibility with the Prison Service which reaches beyond mere compromise to a position where the therapeutic community prison is accommodated within the wider penal structure while yet preserving its essential difference as an example of a humane prison which effectively manages, as well as treats, the dangerous, the disruptive and the 'untreatable'. But the task can never be achieved to everyone's satisfaction. What can be achieved is a clear demonstration by the governor that he/she has an awareness of the issues which matter, including an understanding of their significance to different members, and is prepared to address these issues, however contradictory, in an open and honest way and by endless consultation. It remains a tall, and perhaps impossible, order because there are always those who complain that they have not been consulted, or have not been consulted enough.

The governor as broker

The middleman or broker is another type which has received attention in the anthropological literature. The broker is a key social performer in as much as he/she has special qualifications and competences which enable him/her to operate in two domains. The broker is highly valued because it is through him or her that different groupings are able to engage in a positive relationship. Typically, brokers are merchants, translators, neutral agents and other kinds of go-betweens, who transcend two worlds but belong fully to neither. Their power rests on their ability to benefit or to be seen to benefit, both sides.

I am not suggesting here that as governor of Grendon I act out a formally acknowledged role as broker, rather the position is an informal one that emerges from my structural positioning between the therapeutic community and the overarching Service. Simply to locate myself in a management line somewhere between the prison officer and the Director General would be an oversimplification. On the one hand, I am invested with the responsibility of implementing Prison Service policy and practice while simultaneously pre-serving a therapeutic tradition which may be perceived as being under constant threat. On the other hand, I see my job as promoting Grendon among those who have little understanding of its workings, ranging from those who are friends and supporters to those who are openly critical of what they regard as its radical, eccentric and resource-intensive regime.

I can best illustrate my point by summarising an ongoing tension between therapy and security.

A year before my arrival, the escape of three prisoners from a sports-field had caused a serious setback in confidence over the future of Grendon. An investigation revealed serious flaws in security and rumours circulated about the demise of Grendon as a therapeutic prison. Uncertainty was prolonged when the newly appointed governor left after some five months. There followed an over-long interregnum.

I have described elsewhere how a sense of impending loss was exacerbated by my arrival in September 2002, which coincided with a thorough search of the establishment brought on by the 'discovery' of an electric drill in a prisoner's cell (Bennett, in press). The incident was quite bizarre, not only because some staff and prisoners amazingly failed to see that the possession of such a potential escape implement by a prisoner was a breach of security, but also because searchers clearly overreacted, removing personal items from prisoners' cells which left many of the latter feeling that Grendon had reverted to a 'System' prison. For many, the new governor was the villain of the piece, heralding the final encroachment of an apparent oppressive and brutal penal regime.

The incident brought home to me that the governor had a pivotal role to play in balancing therapy with the needs of security, of ensuring that damaging escapes should be prevented by implementing procedures which would cause minimum damage to the therapeutic regime.

An opportunity arose some months later with the loss of an implement from one of the community kitchens. The normal course of action in a Category B prison would have been to lock prisoners away and to conduct a full search of every cell and association area. But it was clear that a disruptive intervention of this kind could only serve to damage further prisoner–staff relationships, particularly following the traumatic events already described. Values of trust, individual responsibility and openness, intrinsic to the therapeutic process, had already taken a battering. It is in this context that I decided to avoid a typical operational response and to work within therapeutic principles. Having consulted therapists, I personally attended a community meeting and shared with the members my concerns about the breach in security. The experience was not an easy one: prisoners challenged my motives, as well as my previous actions. But they also agreed as a community that the breach of security was indeed of concern and requested that they first be allowed to conduct a search themselves. They found nothing, but nor did the subsequent search by staff. But the episode was something of a breakthrough, an example of how security measures could be implemented while simultaneously acknowledging the values of trust, openness, consultation and enquiry intrinsic to the therapeutic community.

It is significant that not long afterwards, in early 2003, the establishment received a 'good' marking in the national security audit, and had begun to develop a unique cycle of communication between security and the therapeutic communities applauded by the Chief Inspector of Prisons in her report (HMCIoP, 2004). As I write we plan to set up a prisoner Security Committee to report to the main prison Security Committee. This may appear to some to be yet another eccentric idea to emerge from Grendon. And yet it simply acknowledges that most prisoners have a vested interest in maintaining their own security as well as the security of the prison. Grendon may well have accommodated to the overarching structure, but it still retains some of its core values and is still capable of innovation.

Concluding remarks

I have described in some detail, and perhaps rather too self-consciously, how I see my role as governor of Grendon. Given Grendon's unique and ambiguous positioning within the encapsulating Prison Service, the informal nature of the governor's role as broker can be both frustrating and difficult. But governing Grendon in a changing world, while attempting to remain true to the core principles which underpin the therapeutic tradition, is a fascinating and worthwhile challenge. Equality of treatment, care, democratic decision-making, respect for the individual, peer support, openness, consultation, enquiry and welfare are principles which combine to form a distinctive penal tradition which embodies a special and precious expression of humanity.

References

Bennett P (1991) Hull Special Unit. In: K Bottomley and W Hay (eds) *Special Units for Difficult Prisoners.* Centre for Criminology and Criminal Justice, University of Hull.
Bennett P (1993) *The Path of Grace: temple organisation and worship in a Vaishnava sect.* Hindustan Publishing Corporation, Delhi.
Bennett P (in press). Governing Grendon Prison's Therapeutic Communities: the big

spin. In: M Parker (ed) *Dynamic Security : the democratic therapeutic community in prison.* Jessica Kingsley, London.

Clay J (2001) *Maconochie's Experiment.* John Murray, London.

Genders E and Player E (1995) *Grendon: a study of a therapeutic prison.* Oxford University Press, Oxford.

HM Prison Service (2004) MQPL Survey carried out at HMP Grendon between 5 and 9 April 2004 (unpublished).

Her Majesty's Chief Inspector of Prisons for England and Wales (HMCIoP) (2004) *HM Prison Grendon: report on a full inspection 1–5 March 2004.* Home Office, London.

Liebling A (assisted by Arnold H) (2004) *Prisons and their Moral Performance: a study of values, quality and prison life.* Oxford University Press, Oxford.

Niebuhr HR (1929) *The Social Sources of Denominationalism.* Henry Holt, Gloucester, MA.

Troeltsch E (1950) *The Social Teaching of The Christian Churches* (trans. Wyon O). Macmillan, New York, NY.

Weber M (1947) *The Theory of Social and Economic Organization* (trans. Henderson AM and Parsons T). The Free Press, New York, NY.

Wheatley P (2005) Managerialism in the Prison Service. *Prison Service Journal.* **161**(September): 33–4.

Woolf H, Lord Justice and Tumin S Judge (1991) *Prison Disturbances April 1990: report of an inquiry by the Rt Hon Lord Justice Woolf (parts I and II) and His Honour Judge Stephen Tumin (part II).* HMSO, London.

Chapter 12

Clinical supervision for staff in a Therapeutic Community prison

Liz McLure

It is eleven o'clock in the morning; the therapy groups have finished for the day. The staff then meet together for one hour to begin to share and process the five groups they have just facilitated. Each day someone donates a packet of biscuits to the cause. The team bicker and jibe each other in a humorous way over who has the most biscuits, who brought them last, who never brings them, who brought the special chocolate ones. Some are self-sufficient and bring their own sustenance, maintaining difference, not trusting others to feed them properly and resistant to joining in the melée. This is symbolic of the need for nurture and soothing, the hidden aggression and tension, the tremendous drain on individual internal resources and the competition for each to feel special and have their fill in the limited time available. We eventually settle, a new order is found each day and the team begins the business of digesting the morning's events.

Facilitating groups is a complex and complicated process. We have to keep the stories of eight people, their past, their current lives and their relationships in the community and their patterns of relating in mind. We also have to consider the various combinations and connections in the dynamics of the group; this includes the stage of development and history of the group, and the group in the context of the larger therapeutic community (TC) and society at large. There is the need to pay attention to various psychological theories to inform the appropriateness and timing of interventions which may explore, clarify or facilitate the group process. It is necessary to keep in mind one's own story, identifications, blocks, transference and countertransference and to use this in listening to and observing the communications which resonate in the group, some of which are unconscious. Learning about all of this and working with it is the main aim of supervision (McLure, 2000).

Each group is described in turn and thinking about it begins. Themes for each group are then linked and related to community events and incidents. These can be explored and all the pieces of the puzzle can be seen more clearly. What is talked about in one group can give clues to understanding another. Common descriptions of groups are: heavy, like pulling teeth, manic, horrendous, painful, noisy, depressing, powerful, war zone. Staff who have had a difficult group either sit back shellshocked, or demand more time; some hog the space as they cannot bear to take on any more from other groups on top of their own burden. We have tears, tantrums, laughter and sheer desperation. At times when sexual tension and frustration is high on the wing the staff group are flirtatious and playful, the battle of the sexes and an engagement in something that the prisoners are excluded from is played out in this space. Destructiveness and despair is turned into creativity and hope. Staff are allowed free rein to reconnect and offload the feelings that they have had to detach from or contain in order to facilitate the group. 'I could just slap him', 'Oh, he's my baby', 'I'm glad he's not mine', 'I feel sick.' All signifiers of the countertransference, the individual unconscious reactions to the men and their material.

There is never sufficient time to process everything but this meeting is only one part of the supervision process and offers immediate containment of the staff group. The staff then have to switch to the duties required of them in their officer role. They attend to the prison routine, exercise, lunch, work parties, classes, visits, searches, movements. This is necessary to keep the external boundary that the prison offers intact and safe. The therapeutic role is not undermined by this as therapy takes place 24 hours a day, seven days a week. All events and interactions are grist for the therapeutic mill. (This is no excuse for bad behaviour by staff, of course, who can be held accountable in the same way as prisoners.) Thus the staff can easily become conflicted in trying to maintain both functions of their role as well as 'be themselves' in the TC. The task of dynamic administration in maintaining the 'therapeutic space' is often challenged by the inmates and the prison 'system' which is both an internalised structure and externally imposed on the staff. It is often considered remarkable that this regime works, given what is done and who it is done with. Yet all who participate in the therapeutic process are committed to making it work. The nature of the work and the content of the material presented to staff is unbearable (McLure, 2004). Bearing witness to stories of abuse, neglect, cruelty, abandonment, loss, rape, murder, robberies and self-destruction is bad enough. The men present as both the victim and perpetrator in these stories. This is compounded by repetitions of old patterns of behaviour and relationships being acted out. Most offences were committed in states of high arousal, either sexual, aggressive or both combined. Men facing the reality of their internment can return to these states very easily. In therapy there is often the need to take things to the edge, this time not to cross over the boundary and commit an act but to come back and gain understanding of what has happened. In doing this it is possible to unravel the build-up to their arriving in that position. This is a frightening prospect for both the men and staff. It is an emotional rollercoaster, both exciting and terrifying. The complex psychopathology of the men is difficult to tolerate, let alone treat (Mishan and Bateman, 1994).

Staff have a weekly 'sensitivity meeting' where they can share their views on events and interactions in the community. This is an extension of the feedback session described above but also allows staff the space to discuss the experience of pressure from one another and from management. Such pressures can severely test a staff member who is already struggling to cope and who is aware of the heavy burden of responsibility that goes with the work. The difficulties faced by each member of staff is discussed and there is an opportunity to observe for dependency, scapegoating, pairing, splitting and manipulation. All these are signs of a group in distress and unable to function in the task (Bion, 1961). Staff morale can be measured and these phenomena can be explored and given an airing to aid the repair of the staff group. A parallel process can develop which is not always a result of the prisoner's pathology but the other way round: staff regression can re-evoke primitive defences in the men and if not addressed a circular process with increasing regression in both groups can occur (Voorhoeve and van Putte, 1994).

Formal theoretical input and training in preparation for uniformed staff working in this way in prisons can be minimal. In this setting it takes the form of a three-part induction programme in a classroom setting. It often makes little sense to staff until they are immersed in the experience of the work. What they learn in class has to be utilised in supervision and what they learn in practice is given structure and some understanding in the classroom. The theory–practice gap is addressed in this way. Some go on to do an introductory course in group work. This is immensely beneficial to the staff who do complete it since they discover how what they learn is integrated and synthesised with the 'personal self' to be transformed into something that is valuable in the service of the therapeutic work (McLure, 2000).

No amount of theoretical and experiential knowledge alone can prepare anyone for life and work in a TC. The majority of staff will have had no personal therapy prior to undertaking the work and the burden and responsibility of the role of the supervisor is massive as a result of this. Everybody is changed by immersion in this work and the change is not always for the better. Defences are stripped and our own core conflicts exposed in very little time. If a member of staff is not prepared for this event the result can be catastrophic. DW Winnicott put it this way:

> . . . pressing demands of patients for a symbiotic relationship require that facilitators, like mothers with new babies, be able to reach this heightened state of sensitivity, almost an illness, and to recover from it.
>
> (Winnicott, 1958)

In this type of work there is massive projection and transference of feelings and emotions onto the staff group. Some staff can become lost and risk losing their identity in the larger groups, resulting in psychological damage if not managed properly. It is asking a great deal to expect staff with limited experience of therapy and unresolved personal issues to overcome their own neuroses and function in a therapeutic way without casualties arising. There can be the temptation for a growing dependence on the supervisor to deal with all the anxieties and problems. Supervision can very easily turn into a therapy situation so there is a need for clear differentiation between supervision and therapy. If the member of staff gets something completely wrong either in a therapy group or in supervision, this needs to be addressed properly. Acceptance and tolerance has limits when the prisoner (patient) and others are at risk. There is a need to assess 'whether an error is due to a "dumb spot" or a "blind spot" that is, due to ignorance or a product of neurosis, or both' (Gordon, 1995). Both need some attention but it is more the job of the supervisor to attend to the areas of ignorance or misunderstanding.

At times the difficulty in a group's functioning is located in a member of staff. Newer members may comment, 'Oh, we just talked about the state of the wing,' or 'They moaned about the staff.' They are oblivious to what is really being discussed at the deeper levels of communication within the matrix of the group. The defences that keep them engaged in the conversation at this kind of superficial level increases the lack of trust in them as facilitators. Their inexperience and inadequacy is seen through completely and utterly by the group. Attempts may be made to annihilate them, actions representing a wish arising from fear that the prisoners in their oedipal strivings really do not want to be fulfilled. Despair floods the group and the staff member, and if they then 'cave in' under the psychic beating this is disastrous for the group. It gives them the message that they are too dangerous and damaging to be cared for let alone 'sorted' (cured). Hope gets lost with the 'killed off' member of staff.

Staff seen to be under par find themselves scapegoated, ostracised, denigrated and hated. Those who are being idealised do not often see this and can fall into the split created by the anxiety of the men in search of the 'good enough' staff member. The newer, more 'fragile' and insecure staff often begin to act out within a short space of time, e.g. sickness, volunteering for projects off the wing, going on night duty, volunteering for escort duties, refusing to join in the workings of the community without X, Y and Z. Unresolved countertransference that cannot be spoken about can be somatised and often accounts for increased physical illness in the staff group (Campbell Le Fevre, 1994).

Despite the requirement that all staff should be interviewed by a qualified member of the therapy staff, this does not always happen. Unlike many other TCs, not all of our staff are idealistic and some may have complex motives. Some have other agendas for coming to Grendon, which the men with their vast experience in spotting 'Kangas' (a term for system screws, prison officers) with their ulterior motives (promotion, quiet time, personal therapy), soon expose. The Prison Service, when accepting staff who transfer to this specialised therapy unit, does not always take the responsibility of ensuring that they have the emotional resilience, capacity or correct attitude required to do this work. Casualties are frequent if the staff are not managed, nurtured, cared for and given the opportunity to make sense of their experience and integrate their learning in a way that is tailored and appropriate to them as individuals. Group supervision can be too much of a threat for these shellshocked individuals. They either chose to adopt the predominant culture or resist this, becoming a disabling and disabled member of the group.

In group supervision, such as in the feedback sessions, all staff may freely associate to the material. This requires the staff member to have 'the courage of his own stupidity' (Peddar, 1986) to participate in this type of group. For some of the less experienced, vulnerable members of staff, it is too threatening and infantilising. If previous learning experiences involved being punished, humiliated or denigrated in front of others it is easier not to put oneself forward for fear of ridicule. This is a hard obstacle to overcome and the position of learner is felt as a narcissistic blow to be defended by secrecy and obscurity (Fleming and Benedek, 1966). The style of the Prison Service and the expectation that poor performance will result in disciplinary action also makes it difficult to own up to any vulnerability or weakness.

Groups by their nature have a regressive pull and can result in disintegration in the individual to an extent, making it easier to challenge old or to introject new material. This regression can, however, be problematic in this setting as there is no control over what is taken in. The staff may take on board the problems and traumas of the men as if they were their own. This exposure can result in vicarious traumatisation if each event is not satisfactorily processed (Pearlman and Saakvitne, 1995). Without the benefit of their own therapy, the process has to be explained at the same time as it is being used. If their anxiety throws them into crisis it is very difficult to accept new learning about what they are experiencing. If left they may identify with the men, internalise the same maladaptive defensive structures and act out in hostile and destructive ways that are alien to them and counterproductive to the aims of the TC.

If staff view their reactions to the material or changes in their behaviour as shameful or disgusting they will not openly discuss this in front of colleagues/managers. The recognition that we are never that far removed from those we treat in terms of madness or badness is hard to acknowledge – our own potential to harm others is ever-present and frightening. Thus the need is recognised to provide an opportunity for individual support to enable reintegration, understanding and normalisation of their experience in a more contained and supportive setting.

Individual sessions are critical for the newer and less experienced officers who are 'on the fringe' of therapy. They are not fully integrated into the community straight away in that they do not sit on all the small groups. They never facilitate a group on their own until ready to do so. They are, however, still in the firing line of the men who are disturbed and upset when they come out of groups and need someone to discharge their emotions and feelings into.

The qualified therapy staff are used to having clinical supervision but this was not always the culture or expectation of the officers. They had to be actively encouraged to participate. There was resistance initially from some 'more experienced' individuals and attempts at sabotage from the central detailing office (e.g. staff would be reassigned at short notice). Some may have seen it as a 'put down', working from arrogance or ignorance of what supervision entailed, or may have acted on their envy of those in therapy. Setting appointments to meet never worked out. Competing hierarchical structures and the powerful coercive elements of the system were exercised to thwart these. Thus a more loose scheduling arrangement was agreed between the senior officers and the therapy staff. It is now the accepted norm that supervision with me, for example, is on Friday afternoons. Any staff on shift can be invited to attend for one hour each or they can request this for themselves. Like all new ventures, once some see the benefit and value of this space and time with its opportunity to offload and think about the work in relation to themselves, they all want to participate. Indeed new staff now demand to know what it is about and when they will have supervision.

In sessions we work from the known to the unknown. We explore identifications and similarities and then differences in their personal relationships to those of the men. Then we explore the interrelationship between the two. This enables the development of empathy and the objectivity required to tolerate a variety of lifestyles and behaviours. We explore feelings and emotions to the material and think about our reactions to this. We explore our thoughts and feelings around the relationship we have with the men and the groups, and sort out if this belongs to me, or them, or is something between the two that may be important to be fed back into the group. We chat about their families and how things are going in general to pick up on any changes or behaviours that are occurring at home that may be as a result of this work. I say 'we' in all of this as I have discovered that sharing minimises the notion that I am not affected by the work and emphasises that being qualified does not mean that I know everything and they nothing. The space is open and free to talk about anything and everything that may be troubling them.

Psychotherapy in forensic settings is considered to work towards increased suffering in the patients and reduce acting out (Welldon, 1984). With the staff group we try to reduce their suffering and encourage acting in through talking – in supervision, in feedback groups and to one another.

There are some notable differences in the way the male and female staff relate to working in the TC. Female staff have a particularly difficult time as they work in a male prison and the majority of staff are male. They experience different psychological pressures and demands in the therapy situation. The projections and transferences related to all things 'female' can be difficult to contain and even harder to explain to those who will never experience or understand this. The primary relationship with mother is reactivated along with all the manifestations and perversions of this (Madonna, whore and witch). The 'group as mother' can fulfil a basic need for care, nurture and responsiveness to each individual. However, without an actual female, aspects of difference in gender and the opportunity to explore the development of sexual relatedness at a profound level is missing. Men can, of course, rekindle and connect with their early maternal relationship and engage with this to care for others, but for those who had no experience of the 'good enough mother' (unfortunately most of our men) this aspect remains absent from the group without a female member. The groups without a female facilitator tend to be more aggressive and abusive towards each other. Those with a female are envied and attacked by those without. There is great competition and rivalry for the attention of female staff, which makes them more vulnerable to all the attacks that arise from the above. There is also great fear of attachment to and dependence on females that is coupled with envy, rage and hatred when the men are invariably disappointed in not getting what they need and want from the staff.

The special position of women

Although the community attempts to represent a microcosm of society there are no female peers for the prisoners. Thus the female staff can be pulled more towards sharing intimate information about themselves. Some have gone too far in this and shared their difficulties in relationships and talked of their sex lives to the men. Sexual contact is forbidden, which can reactivate the incest taboo. Some female members of staff struggle with this and adopt unusual behaviours to either hide or emasculate their femininity. They may dress in dowdy dark clothes in an attempt to deny their gender. Some identify with the misogynistic parts of themselves internalised from other relationships, and attack their femininity by becoming 'one of the boys', cutting their hair short and adopting crude self-effacing language. Others are lulled into using their sexuality to seduce or be seduced in an attempt to retain or regain position and the control that is perceived as lost. Some, when challenged about getting too close to breaking the boundaries, perceive this as an envious attack from the other female staff. They often do not see this as caring for them and the men and may act out and engage in sexual relationships. This not only damages each individual but compromises the whole community. Those who are secure in their femininity are able to provide the non-sexual mirroring that the men require in the further development of their self-concept and -esteem.

Relationships at home can suffer if staff become preoccupied and all-consumed by the work. Those who have difficulty in external relationships and have low self-esteem are more easily psychologically enticed into the role of loving parent. This is a powerfully seductive scenario in which the staff member experiences the gratification of being loved and may develop fantasies of receiving the patient's undying gratitude, confirming of their own sense of worth (Cox, 1980). Women know how powerful an infant can be and the temporary sacrifice of the self in that dyad. The risk of merger with the madness of the unintegrated, regressed individual is a real threat to her. Female staff are often more able to express their own emotional reactions and their receptivity to the emotional states of the men in therapy. The men are also very sensitive to the emotional states and vulnerabilities of the female staff and readily project their vulnerability into them when in this state. They are both threatened and reassured by the female staff. The fact that most survive whatever the community throws at them is the source of their power.

Ambiguous position of male staff

Male staff tend to be a bit more pragmatic. On the surface they appear to be less emotional and expend a great deal of energy in 'provision' of practical things to make life more comfortable (for all). This image of the father figure who is in control and has authority and purpose is emulated by most male staff. They compete with each other for the title of leader or best provider. If they come to depend on this position to boost their self-worth and value, this can result in a regressive dependence on them from the men and a bigger burden is then placed upon them to continue in the role of 'saviour'. Those with experience and confidence are able to show their 'female' qualities and see this as a strength. To lose face and be endowed with 'female' qualities is a threat for the less secure, especially in a prison. They defend against feelings of impotence, inadequacy and failure; they do not wish to be so exposed in front of the men they are expected to control and take charge of, men who have already demonstrated their prowess (and inadequacy) in their offences. The men are always in competition with the male staff. Some staff get heavily involved in the authoritarian aspects of their split role, becoming rule-bound and harsh, widening the 'them and us' split between the staff and men. They may struggle with expression of love and care as well as responsibility towards the men. Homophobic reactions may surface as a defence against this closeness and the development of secure male bonding with appropriate boundaries. 'Banter' and macho posturing tends to disguise much of this. The 'system' also adds to the difficulty in developing trust in the perverse insistence that the male staff carry out the mandatory 'strip searches' that accompany the frequent drug testing and cell searches on the wing. This raises real anxiety and disgust in staff and the men, particularly with those who are working through experiences of being sexually abused as children. The staff need to talk about this and how they can be sensitive in the way this procedure is carried out. They can feel like abusers and can hate themselves and those who say they must do it; conversely some may gain satisfaction in exercising control and humiliating another in this way. This too has to be picked up and talked about. These experiences, like any other, provide opportunities for developing greater empathy and understanding of the men; the effects of violation of another can be explored from all perspectives.

The men in the community are aware that staff have supervision; they too see it as beneficial and alert us if they feel that staff are struggling to cope, such is their respect for and willingness to reciprocate in the care and concern for those who are here to care for them.

For supervision to become a suitable transformational space or place to play and explore we have to encourage the staff to be honest in their feedback of mistakes, faults and lack of skills in some areas:

> We can and do learn a great deal from our mistakes. It should offer greater opportunity for aesthetic moments or unprocessed connections to be made as there is always more than meets the eye going on in the community. It is essential to help them to discern and address emotional states which, if unrecognised and unaddressed, interfere with the task of the therapy and ignore the learning and understanding that is available from every interaction.
>
> (Behr, 1995)

Supervision is not therapy, yet at times it is necessary to help a member of staff to cope with a personal dilemma that is interfering with their ability to function and encourage them to take responsibility for that part of their own mental hygiene. Staff, like community members, stay on a wing for years at a time. Thus, how they cope with life events and crises is observed by the community. To deny that something is affecting a member of staff would confuse the men's experience of them when they pick up the change in the way the staff member is relating. However, it is neither necessary nor helpful for the whole community to know details of staff's personal struggles. There are times when staff are given time out to deal with a raw issue before returning to work on the community. Their vulnerability would affect their ability to contain the therapy for the men. We often find that, when staff are discovered to be human and take time to seek help to sort themselves out rather than damage relationships, this is admired and respected by the men who struggle to cope with their own emotional worlds.

Work influence on family relationships

Many changes in the staff can be observed in their interactions with each other and in the community. Unfortunately there are times when the material they are presented with is carried home and they may begin to behave uncharacter-istically or change in their relationships with family and friends. Dads may no longer bathe or hug their children for fear of abusing them, women go off sex and hate their partners, seeing them as rapists. Men or women may neglect or beat their partners or children, become strict and controlling at home. Some become hyper-vigilant and withdraw from social interactions, and depression can set in. These are all signs of vicarious traumatisation (Pearlman and Saakvitne, 1995). The links with the work and the displacement of their thoughts and feelings needs to be acknowledged and explored in supervision to avoid permanent damage to their relationships. At times the staff member listening on the group comes to realise that their way of being is damaging to their families; thus change in them can be positive and beneficial too.

The psychopathology of the staff group also needs careful consideration. If their pre-morbid personality (prior to working on the TC) was unstable and they got beaten up or into fights regularly, are dependent on alcohol or drugs, or cannot maintain relationships, they are very vulnerable. Feelings of inadequacy, guilt and shame surrounding their own lack of control are amplified and will paralyse them emotionally in the community. They will either be unable to challenge this in others or will massively project and abuse those in their care. Those with low self-esteem will invariably, in order to be liked and accepted, unconsciously identify and collude with the men to avoid incurring their rage. They break boundaries, both physical (leaving gates open) and psychological in that they lie, divulge staff information and break confidences; they become compromised and this is extremely dangerous in a prison setting. They are enticed into collusion with the anti-group in its perversion of what is good and bad (Mishan and Bateman 1994). Those staff who are unwell mentally with poor ego functioning will inevitably disinte-grate and break down. Manic defences against anxiety are not uncommonly observed – obsessive cleaning, joking and making fun of every situation are the most frequent indicators of this. Taking on the 'system' and deliberately breaking rules using the men as pawns and encouraging them to 'take sides' as they play the victim is more serious. Those who flee from the experience, become abusive, or disengage and dissociate totally from the material replay the men's core conflicts and situations where parents were absent, neglectful, abusive or deranged mentally. The men's transferences and projections are soaked up and eventually when the staff member does break down, the opportunity to process what happened is lost. All of this has to be explored and managed in the therapy for the men and the supervision for the staff. Staff need the time it takes to grow and change. Ordinarily they are allowed to reach the stage of readiness to accept new knowledge and accommodate; this is not normally forced or insisted upon. However, supervisors have to challenge resistance to change in the staff. Time is precious to those who are 'doing time' – they cannot afford to wait for staff to become good enough, they need staff who can function with sufficient integrity and self awareness to be effective in sharing this dangerous journey with them.

The provision of clinical supervision is both necessary and problematic, as in all TCs containment of the staff improves the functioning of the commu-nity – without containment we would all flounder and would be less able to do the seemingly impossible and hopefully improve the quality of life of the men we care for. This is the ideal and we have also to face up to the reality that those men who return to the community still have the potential to cause serious harm or even death. This is a burden no one takes lightly: it is the constant shadowy fear in the background of our mind (Choma, 1998).

References

Behr H (1995) The integration of theory and practice. In: M Sharpe (ed) *The Third Eye: supervision of analytic groups*. Routledge, London.

Bion WR (1961) *Experiences in Groups*. Tavistock, London.

Campbell Le Fevre D (1994) The power of countertransference in groups for the severely mentally ill. *Group Analysis*. **27**: 441–7.

Choma MW (1998) Commentary on Weiss paper: Some reflections on countertransference in the treatment of criminals. *Psychiatry*. **61**: 178-180.

Cox M (1980) Cited in: M Meinrath and JP Roberts (2004) On being a good enough staff member. *Therapeutic Communities*. **25**(4): 318–24.

Fleming J and Benedek TF (1966, reprinted 1983) *Psychoanalytic Supervision. a method of clinical teaching*. Grune & Stratton, New York, NY.

Gordon RM (1995) The symbolic nature of the supervisory relationship: identification and professional growth. *Issues in Psychoanalytic Psychology*. **17**: 154–62.

McLure E (2000) *The contribution of Group Analytic Principles to an understanding of how students synthesize theory, personal therapy and practice on a Group Analytic Psychotherapy Training Course*. Unpublished MSc thesis, University of Sheffield.

McLure E (2004) Working with the unbearable. In: D Jones (ed) *Working With Dangerous People*. Radcliffe Medical Press, Oxford.

Mishan J and Bateman A (1994) Group analytic therapy in borderline patients in a day hospital setting. *Group Analysis*. **27**: 483–95.

Peddar J (1986) Reflections on the theory and practice of supervision. *Psychoanalytic Psychotherapy*. **2**(1): 1–12.

Pearlman LA and Saakvitne KW (1995) *Trauma and the Therapist: countertransference and vicarious traumatisation in psychotherapy with incest survivors*. WW Norton Professional, New York, NY.

Voorhoeve JN and van Putte FCA (1994) 'Parallel Process' in supervision when working with psychotic patients. *Group Analysis*. **27**: 459–46.

Welldon E (1984) Application of Group Analytic Psychotherapy to those with sexual perversons. In: Lear T (ed) *Spheres of Group Analysis*. GAS Publications, London.

Winnicott DW (1958) *Through Paediatrics to Psychoanalysis*. Hogarth Press, London.

Chapter 13

Psychotherapy in prisons: a supervisor's view

Tilman Kluttig

The focus of this paper is on psychotherapeutic practice in the German prison system from a supervisor's perspective. It was Murray Cox (1996) who made the essential statement at the beginning of his paper on supervision in forensic psychotherapy in the most elaborated volume on forensic psychotherapy from Cordess and Cox (1996) that:

> The first thing to say about supervision is that it is, or should be, sine qua non of all forensic therapeutic undertakings.
>
> (Cordess and Cox, 1996, p. 199)

His argument is that the difficult and even perilous work of forensic psychotherapists and institutions needs professional supervision to enable secure treatment for offenders' psychopathology. Following this point supervision has to be a part of the treatment setting – it is necessary that supervision is guaranteed

> . . . before the therapeutic wheels begin to turn . . .
>
> (*ibid.*, p. 199)

Supervision in forensic treatment settings and in the prison services has a plurivalent character. First of all supervision should be helpful for the therapeutic endeavour of patients and therapists. Here the function of supervision is to help understand the meaning of transference and countertransference in the therapeutic relationship and to process embarrassing, seducing, humiliating, hurting or sadistic material which is presented by the offender and may shock or frighten the therapist. Especially in the prison setting the supervisor is often asked about aspects of prognostic assessment. Therapists have a legitimate interest in refining their treatment interventions or further decision-making about the prisoner by discussing them in supervision and having them supported by the professional authority of the supervisor. This part of supervision in prisons is often close to the meaning of supervision as control, ensuring that therapy is done the right way in order to be protected from the charge of deficient work if any critical incident happens. So, supervision in forensic settings seems to be more broadly based than it may be in other therapeutic settings and this also mirrors the differences between forensic psychotherapy and general psychotherapy.

As far as I can evaluate it for the German prison system the way in which supervision for psychotherapists working in prisons is provided is not at all appropriate to Cox's postulation above. A survey on the German 'therapeutic prison system', the so-called 'Sozialtherapie' (social therapy), shows that even in these special prisons supervision is only partly integrated in the treatment setting. In 2005, 40 per cent of these institutions offered supervision for therapists, and – a more respectable number – 84.4 per cent supervision for treatment teams (Kriminologische Zentralstelle, 2005). But this covers only a small part of the German prison system.

A neglected aspect of supervisory work in the prison system is beyond the treatment aspect. In exploring the relationships and dynamics of prisoners and staff, supervisory or counselling work could contribute to coping with the difficult life behind bars.

The following ideas result from several years in which I have had the privilege to be supervisor of colleagues doing their often difficult work as psychotherapists in the German prison system.

Psychotherapy in German prisons

German criminal justice has essentially a double-tracked system of prison sentences and commitment to treatment in forensic psychiatry or an institution for withdrawal treatment (Volckart, 1999). Treatment in forensic psychiatry requires as a precondition that the court found the offender not criminally liable or with reduced liability at the time of the offence for reasons of mental illness (which can include personality disorders and paraphilias) and that there is certain risk of ongoing danger to the public without treatment. Treatment in an institution for withdrawal treatment requires a close connection between offences and an addictive disorder, and a certain prospect that treatment might be successful.

In 2004 in Germany, about 81 000 people were imprisoned in 203 penal institutions in Germany (Jehle, 2005). At the end of 2004, Germany's population was approximately 82 500 000. In 2005, 1682 prisoners were treated in the above-mentioned special prisons, the 'Sozialtherapie' (Kriminologische Zentralstelle, 2005).

Psychotherapeutic treatment in prisons aims for the treatment of psychological disorders and mental illnesses on the one hand, and on the other hand for rehabilitation of the offender. As in other countries, we can identify a group with psychological problems in the prison population. For example, Frädrich and Pfäfflin (2000) analysed a representative sample of the German prison population and could find a prevalence of 50 per cent of personality disorders, mainly cluster B type. In another study, Blocher et al. (2001) carried out an investigation with the symptom checklist (SCL-90) of Derogatis. More than half of the prison population showed severe psychopathological symptoms – compared with healthy controls the amount of psychic stress was three times as high. They found mainly dysphoric and depressive symptoms, suicidal tendencies and paranoid thinking.

The treatment of violent and sex offenders had always been within the domain of psychotherapeutic treatment in the prison system. After a series of severe sexual crimes (some of the offenders had previous prison sentences for sexual offences or had just been released from the prison system) a new law was passed in 1998, the law for the abatement of sexual crime and other severe offences. In addition to the fact that this law tightened up the prognostic criteria informing court decisions for the release of these offenders, it imposed an obligation on violent and sex offenders with prison sentences over two years at least to start a psychotherapeutic treatment when this was indicated. The idea was that these treatments should mainly be performed in the 'Sozialtherapie' but nevertheless other prisons started special treatment programmes as well, mostly cognitive behavioural in approach. A positive side-effect was that all German states started programmes for the qualification of therapists in prison and supervision was now more easily available for prison psychotherapists. Nevertheless, there is still a gap between the demands claimed by this law and a lack of treatment places.

Treatment in the 'sozialtherapie' has a tradition in the German prison system. The first institution was a prison near Stuttgart, a former fortress and a prison of the Dukes and Kings of Württemberg, the Hohenasperg. Here in 1954, Gerhard Mauch developed the principles of social therapy. His conception was that social therapy should help the offender to move from a criminal group or culture to a social group or culture. A modified psychodynamic therapy integrating guidance, counselling, educational elements and social work was the essence of this conception (Mauch and Mauch, 1969). In the coming years social therapeutic institutions integrated elements from therapeutic communities and from milieu therapy and developed a structured treatment approach with differentiated concepts for admission, treatment phase, release phase and aftercare (Egg, 1985).

Psychological services are today a common feature of prisons delivering psychotherapeutic treatment and psychometric and prognostic assessment. Treatment programmes for sex offenders or special training for violent offenders are common practice, but availability of continuous and intense psychotherapeutic treatment is still rare. In small prisons due to a lack of qualified staff psychotherapeutic work might be done by colleagues outside the prison's staff.

General parameters of psychotherapy in prisons

Psychotherapists in prison have to be aware of some basic parameters determining the therapeutic process. First of all, and this is a specific feature of forensic psychotherapy in contrast to general psychotherapy, the therapy takes place not in the total privacy of the psychotherapeutic consulting room but under the vigilant eyes of the public, the judiciary and the institution. To mention this seems to be trivial and a lot has already been written about it, but nevertheless it is important in the supervisory process: to neglect this can lead to fatal misjudgment and entanglement of the psychotherapist and seriously interfere with his work. The prison environment and setting can be a place where a re-enactment of violence and of dynamics of offending and being victimised can easily happen. Our psychotherapeutic undertakings with offenders have always to relate the here-and-now experience and behaviour of the offender patient with the criminal act:

> . . . the arena in which forensic psychotherapy is undertaken demands all that is
> expected of generic dynamic psychotherapy with the crucial codicil that the

> highest discriminatory attention is also paid to the context. This is important because it links the here-and-now of present dynamic engagement with the there-and-then of the past dynamic engagement in which the criminal act took place.
>
> (Cox, 1996, pp. 204 f)

A well known stereotype in forensic psychotherapy is the concept of cultures struggling against each other in prisons: criminal culture versus therapeutic culture, with conflicting values concerning, for example offending, behaviour and expression of emotions (Doctor, 1997). Hinshelwood (1996) described this dynamic as a clash between care versus toughness culture and described elements of this from the perspectives of the prison staff and the prisoners. He emphasised this as well as an important expression of the need to belong to a group. Here we have to understand that in forensic psychotherapy we have to recognise that treatment often starts on the part of the prisoners with the question of who is on his side rather than with the idea of neutrality. Prisoners (and sometimes prison staff) usually want to know if the therapist is 'on their side' or if he is on the side of the adversary, the prison system (Pecher, 2002). They are trying to 'use' the therapist in a way which may be abusive or can be misunderstood as abusive:

> Prisoners' fears and neediness are immediately converted into a trickery that can assert a superiority and independence over the person of whom the demand is being made.
>
> (Hinshelwood, 1996, p. 470)

This phenomenon is on both sides – therapist and prisoner – an important trigger for transference processes. The therapist can be seen by the prisoner as a powerful and dominating representative of the punishing system or as a friendly and helpful person, protecting the prisoner against the unjust prison system. Countertransference reactions of therapists might be identification with the power of the institution or – more often – feelings of helplessness or impotence (Pecher, 2002). It is clear that to work on this dynamic is crucial to avoid a malignant and unrealistic splitting.

In close relationship with the above-mentioned points is a discussion of motivational issues. Of course the evaluation of motivation for therapeutic treatment is an important point, especially if the resources for offering psychotherapy are limited. The concept of motivation often seems not very clear and hardly operationalised. Sometimes a neutral observer could have the idea that the evaluation of motivation of a prisoner for therapy might be more an expression of the motivation of the therapist to work with a certain patient or prisoner than of the prisoner's own motivation.

In my supervisory work, I have the impression that here the concepts of motivation have changed in recent years in a constructive way. In particular, developments in the treatment of addictive disorders and severe personality disorders have been helpful in recognising that motivation is not a static concept but a dynamic process which can be influenced and developed to a certain degree by therapeutic interventions. In his research of the German prison system, Dahle (1995) demonstrates that motivation for 'psychotherapy behind bars' (the title of his book) is an ambiguous construct linked to process. Therapists have to face different groups of prisoners and to think about differential strategies to help develop a motivation for psychotherapy in prisoners. In his study he identified several groups of prisoners with different motivations.

- One group felt responsible for their situation, felt not very stressed by their social situation and had no or only few problems in accepting and using therapy or other services of the prison, e.g. professionally qualified support.
- Another group felt not at all responsible, had a style of external attribution and had severe prejudices against therapy and the prison system.
- Another group felt extremely stressed being in prison and by the consequences of their offences. This group was characterised by a feeling of general helplessness, by deficits in the social development, and by severe social burdens in their actual situation. They were interested in therapeutic help but not all able to do anything to get that help.
- Another group felt an extreme strain from being imprisoned and by the consequences of the offence. They had in general positive expectations concerning psychotherapy. Here Dahle identified two subgroups: The first had a positive attitude towards psychotherapy but expected negative influences of the prison situation on the therapeutic process (e.g. privacy, negative evaluation, reactions of other prisoners). The other subgroup had severe doubts as to whether they could stand the therapeutic challenge.

Dahle's results show clearly that motivation, constraint and freedom have to be seen as very complex concepts in forensic psychotherapy (1995, p. 194ff). But we have to keep in mind that constraint as secondary motivation for psychotherapy has to be replaced by positive experiences in the therapeutic setting to develop a mutual working alliance (Kluttig, 2000). Maintaining change requires that patients take responsibility for their own development.

In evaluating motivation we should not forget that there are important differences between offenders who are in prison for the first time, offenders who repeatedly serve sentences and offenders who have been in prison for a very long time already. Especially in the last group we can see that these prisoners often present more of their experiences in imprisonment and the psychological problems connected with it than the initial offence. This sometimes can be easily misunderstood as simple denial but is in fact often a result of coping with the prison situation.

Some patterns of transference and countertransference

I have already mentioned patterns of transference and countertransference resulting from the context of forensic psychotherapy in prison. Of course these patterns are closely connected or mixed with dynamics resulting from specific disorders and/or specific delinquency (Strasburger, 1986; Mintzer, 1996; Meloy, 2002).

In the treatment of antisocial syndromes we have to face therapeutic pessimism resulting from the idea of untreatability of these patients. Their poor capacity in relating, trust, self-observation and self-control often seems to prove this and prompts the therapist to a punishing reaction. A whole part of treatment might be characterised by different ways the patient tries to use 'avenues of escape through action' (Strasberger, 1986, p. 192). It is useful to construct problem areas instead of accepting narcissistic megalomania, complete self-devaluation or the hidden narcissism of a 'desperado identity' who has nothing to lose. Treatment of the antisocial patient needs boundaries and rules, active intervention and the willingness of therapists to give guidance to the patient. The supervisory process is often dominated by the effort of keeping a balance between acting out of the patient and reasonable reactions of the therapist. Feelings of fear are very important. We have to find out:

> . . . how to distinguish between countertransference distortion and prudential fear . . .
>
> (Cox, 1996, p. 205)

otherwise an overrating of dangerousness could lead to unjustified sanctions and destroy the therapeutic work. On the other hand, avoidance or underestimation could lead to prognostically fatal errors. Denial is a common defence mechanism in work with dangerous patients, especially if the therapist identifies with the grandiose self of the patient or has hidden fearful feelings towards him.

We have to be clear that a working alliance with patients with antisocial syndromes is discontinuous and incomplete, therefore Strasberger's concept of problem areas is very helpful. Meloy (2002) warned that one type of countertransference reaction can be the illusion of a existing working alliance.

Patients with antisocial characters are confronting the professional identity of the therapist as a helpful person. They tend to make the therapist responsible and to disprove him – a reaction of the therapist might be to quarrel with the patient, to devaluate him or to feel helpless and impotent. We might have to bear severe feelings of hate and destructiveness. Narcissistic persons are confronting us with an idealisation of their own person and devaluation of others. They may use the therapist as a 'supporter' or 'sparring partner' but not as a significant other. Typical countertransference reactions might be either aggression and protest, or boredom and disinterest.

Especially in the treatment of sex offenders, therapists' transference reactions might be influenced by public discussions. Therapists have to steer clear of the Scylla of identifying with the offenders and the Charybdis of identifying with the idea of sex offender as a stigmatised outsider from society. Feelings like disgust, anger and contempt must be contained, as well as the professional obligation to work with culturally 'dirty' material. Breer (1987) talked about the problem of therapists of sex offenders either becoming 'rescuers' or 'prosecutors'.

Fear, shame, helplessness and uncertainty are common feelings in work with forensic patients, feelings that are opposed to the culture of toughness in prisons and forensic institutions. Therefore, it is important that the supervision session is a helpful and supporting act:

> The threatening supervision session is as great a distortion of what is meant to be a supportive process as a 'staff support group' in which participants are afraid to submit that they need support.
>
> (Cox, 1996, p. 207)

Supervision in the forensic field should meet the needs of the supervisee. As I mentioned at the beginning of this paper, these might go beyond the analysis of transference processes and have to include sometimes support, advice and didactic teaching.

Conclusion and perspectives

Supervision in prisons has to pay very conscientious attention to the complex matrix of societal, institutional and individual dynamics and processes involved in the difficult project of psychotherapy in prisons. The complexity of this and the difference from general psychotherapy makes supervision an imperative element of therapeutic services in the prison system. A helpful guideline on the course of forensic psychotherapy in prison is always to be aware of the actual state of the therapeutic working alliance. Outside the forensic field, transference-focused psychotherapy has been developed for the treatment of borderline personality disorders (Clarkin *et al.*, 2001). Recently Lackinger and Damman (2005) proposed to evaluate whether this approach could be a helpful contribution to the forensic field as well. Though transference-focused psychotherapy was not developed for application to the treatment of offenders, some aspects seem to be helpful and worth being adapted to the forensic field. These include especially the emphasis on the working alliance which does not already exist when therapist and patient meet for the first time. The elaborated concept of establishing a working alliance as a first stage in therapy by transference-focused psychotherapy might provide an example for forensic psychotherapy. It includes transparency by defining the frame of therapy, a clear statement concerning the roles of patient and therapist and an agreement on the responsibilities of therapist and patient in the therapeutic process. Such setting variables seem to be helpful to keep free from the reefs and shallows of unconscious dynamics endangering the therapeutic process. Transference-focused psychotherapy delivers a practical framework for supervision in the forensic field.

Humane prisons need the element of psychotherapy. Not only because of the offer of a treatment service for some prisoners but because psychotherapeutic knowledge and analysis may contribute essentially in the understanding of the complex dynamics of these institutions and help to minimise destructive processes. Here again we can refer to Murray Cox on supervision as a basic necessity of forensic psychotherapy.

References

Blocher D, Henkel K, Ziegler E and Rösler M (2001) Zur Epidemiologie psychischer Beschwerden bei Häftlingen einer Justizvollzugsanstalt. (Epidemiology of psychological disorders in prisoners) *Recht & Psychiatrie*. **19**: 136–40.

Breer W (1987) *The Adolescent Molester*. Thomas, Springfield, IL.

Clarkin JF Yeomans FE and Kernberg OK (2001) *Psychotherapie der Borderline-Persönlichkeit. Manual zur Transference-Focused Psychotherapy* (Psychotherapy for borderline personality. Manual of transference focused psychotherapy). Schattauer, Stuttgart.

Cordess C and Cox M (eds) (1996) *Forensic Psychotherapy: crime, psychodynamics and the offender patient.* Vol. I & II. Jessica Kingsley, London.

Cox M (1996) A supervisor's view. In: C Cordess and M Cox (eds) (1996) *Forensic Psychotherapy: crime, psychodynamics and the offender patient.* Vol. II: Mainly Practice. Jessica Kingsley, London.

Dahle KP (1995) *Therapiemotivation hinter Gittern* (Motivation for psychotherapy behind bars). Roderer, Regensburg.

Derogatis LR. SCL-90-R® Symptom Checklist-90-Revised. www.pearsonassessments.com/tests/scl90r.htm

Doctor R (1997) Abhängigkeit, Sucht und Kriminalität in einer Therapeutischen Gemeinschaft innerhalb des Strafvollzugs (Drug dependency, addiction and crime in a therapeutic community in the prison system). *Recht & Psychiatrie.* **15**: 155–9.

Egg R (1985) *Straffälligekit und Strafvollzug* (The penal system and the convicted). Heymans, Köln.

Frädrich S and Pfäfflin F (2000) Zur Prävalenz von Persönlichkeitsstörungen bei Strafgefangenen (The prevalence of personality disorders in a prison population). *Recht & Psychiatrie.* **18**: 95–104.

Hinshelwood RD (1996) Changing prisons. The unconscious dimension. In: C Cordess and M Cox (eds) (1996) *Forensic Psychotherapy: crime, psychodynamics and the offender patient.* Vol. II: Mainly Practice. Jessica Kingsley, London.

Jehle J (2005) *Criminal Justice in Germany.* Federal Ministry of Justice, Berlin.

Kriminologische Zentralstelle (2005) *Soziatherapie im Strafvollzug* (Social therapy in the prison system). Bearbeitet von K Schulz. Kriminologische Zentralstelle, Wiesbaden.

Kluttig T (2000) Komplexe Behandlungsaufgaben und Behandlungsplanung in der stationären forensischen Psychotherapie (Specialized treatment and treatment planning in forensic psychiatry). *Werkstattschriften Forensische Psychiatrie und Psychotherapie.* **7**: 221–40.

Lackinger F and Damman G (2005) Besonderheiten der Behandlungsbedingungen bei der übertragungsfokussierten Psychotherapie persönlichkeitsgestörter Delinquenten (Transference focused psychotherapy for offenders with personality disorders). *Recht & Psychiatrie.* **23**: 103–15.

Mauch G and Mauch R (1969) Sozialtherapie in der Strafanstalt. Möglichkeiten und Grenzen. (Social therapy in the prison: Potentials and limits) In: W Bitter (ed) *Verbrechen – Schuld oder Schicksal?* (Crime – guilt or fate?) Klett-Cotta, Stuttgart.

Meloy JR (2002) *The Psychopathic Mind: origin, dynamics and treatment.* Jason Aronson, Lanham.

Mintzer MB (1996) Understanding countertransference reactions in working with adolescent perpetrators of sexual abuse. *Bull Menninger Clinic.* **60**(2): 219–28.

Pecher W (2002) Zur Psychodynamik der Institution Strafvollzug (Psychodynamics of prison measures). *Recht & Psychiatrie.* **20**: 63–8.

Strasburger LH (1986) The treatment of antisocial syndromes: the therapist's feelings. In: WH Reid, D Dorr, JI Walker and JW Bonner (eds) *Unmasking the Psychopath: antisocial personality and related syndromes.* Norton, New York, NY.

Volckart B (1999) *Maßregelvollzug. Das Recht des Vollzugs der Unterbringung nach §§ 63, 64 StGB in einem psychiatrischen Krankenhaus und in einer Entziehungsanstalt* (Forensic psychiatry. A comment on the law of commitment following articles 63 and 64 of the penal code to treatment in a psychiatric hospital or an institution for withdrawal treatment) (5e). Luchterhand, Neuwied.

Chapter 14

Peer-review and accreditation

Sarah Tucker and Adrian Worrall

Overview

This chapter shows how a review process grounded in humane values can help develop, safeguard and promote humane prisons. It uses examples from the Community of Communities review process of democratic therapeutic communities in prisons. With particular reference to the good work of HM Inspectorate of Prisons, the chapter first outlines the policy and service context highlighting that there is an outstanding need to:

- promote humane values
- outwardly account for standards of care.

It then shows that therapeutic community prisons:

- are built on these values
- are proven effective even for serious offenders.

It further shows how audit and peer-review provides a cost effective way of not only demonstrating standards of care, but further developing and safeguarding these values. It is argued that monitoring change is intrinsic to the audit and peer-review process and that this is augmented by both celebrating achievements as well as to work on areas for improvement. Following a summary of critical questions concerning this approach and the implications of accreditation, it concludes that a therapeutic community prison regulated by an audit and peer-review provides an ideal model of service.

Policy context and the rise of regulation

The combination of external standard-setting, external standard-monitoring and internal governance systems is the foundation of new British government reforms in health and in other sectors (see, for example, Department of Health, 1997).

New policy was shaped around the urgent need to avoid the scandal and tragedies of the recent past. In the health service in the 1990s, failures in bone tumour diagnosis in Birmingham, cancer screening in Exeter and Kent and paediatric heart surgery in Bristol shocked the public and directly highlighted the serious shortcomings of existing management systems.

A string of corporate scandals such as insider trading (e.g. the Guinness affair of 1987) and pension fund embezzlement (e.g. the Mirror Group in 1991) led to 'corporate governance' being devised as a way to make senior executives more accountable in cases of corporate fraud. 'Clinical governance' was adapted from this. It imposes a statutory duty of quality on NHS organisations and those that lead them (under the Health Act 1999).

The scale and frequency of scandal in the Prison Service is unrivalled in any other public sector service. Following a series of high-profile escapes, in 1995 the Director General of the Prison Service was controversially sacked. There are still regular reports of prison officer brutality (Dodd, 2003), high levels of suicide (Royal College of Psychiatrists, 2002) and homicide (Public Inquiry into the death of Zahid Mubarek, 2000), self-harm and lack of mental health care (HM Inspectorate of Prisons, 2004), racist violence and overcrowding (HM Inspectorate of Prisons, 2005). Overcrowding and consequent large and frequent movement of prisoners around the prison system contribute to high levels of death in prisons (Joint Committee On Human Rights, 2004). Many have pointed out the UK government's responsibility to reduce these deaths by reducing overcrowding (see, for example, Wilson, 2005). The lack of mental healthcare is particularly worrying given the very high prevalence of mental disorders in the prison population (ONS, 1998). Some 'very seriously mentally ill young people' requiring constant observation are held in UK prisons rather than psychiatric hospitals (HMIP, 2005). This makes their conditions worse – it would be hard to imagine a less therapeutic environment than an overcrowded prison.

These profound and serious problems have caused the most senior figures in the prison service to threaten resignation (Travis, 2001), or produce damning reports, books and speeches (see, for example, Ramsbotham, 2003).

Legal framework and regulation

The Prison Act 1952 is the primary legal framework in the UK and it empowers the Minister to make rules for the management of prisons. Many of these rules refer to aims of prison management such as 'treatment and training', the promotion of 'self-respect' and the development of 'personal responsibility' – aims that accord well with humane values. There are also important international human rights instruments, in particular those of the United Nations.

Unfortunately international and national regulations have little impact on the routine management and monitoring of prisons in the UK (Morgan, 2002); for example, the Prison Service annual reports focus primarily on management objectives and performance indicators.

Prisons have standards and an independent regulator but no statutory 'duty of quality' such as clinical governance in the health sector. There is therefore no requirement to have a comprehensive internal system of steps and procedures to monitor and improve the quality of service and thus the tripartite reform model is incomplete. Like other public services, however, prisons are accountable for the quality and safety of their service. They are accountable for public safety – in terms of effective containment during the sentence and also effective reduction in public risk when prisoners are released. They also have a duty to explain to the outside world what happens inside their walls and also the likely outcomes of imprisonment (Coyle, 2002).

These duties are partly achieved by Her Majesty's Inspectorate of Prisons for

England and Wales (HMIP). This was established in 1980 to inspect and report on prisons in England and Wales (*see* Chapter 15). In 2001 the Chief Inspector, Sir David Ramsbotham, produced 'Expectations', a set of standards for the treatment and conditions of prisoners, in response to the shocking conditions of prisons revealed in many reports. Since then, Chief Inspectors' reports based on these objective standards have had more impact on policy (Morgan, 2002).

Now in their second edition, the standards (HMIP, 2004) are based on principles described in the World Health Organization's concept of a healthy prison, of safe, respectful and purposeful treatment of prisoners and their effective resettlement. After inspection, a local report is provided and managers are expected to address its recommendations in an action plan. Every five years each prison receives an inspection and a follow-up visit.

The work of the HMIP is impressive but not sufficient. Fundamental failings in privacy, safety, dignity and duty of care remain widespread in prisons:

> Year after year, governor after governor, inspection after inspection, prisons like these have been exposed. Year after year, the exposure has led to a flurry of hand-wringing, sometimes a change of governor, a dash of capital investment but no real or sustained improvement.
>
> (Travis 2001, quoted in the *Guardian*)

Prisons need support and resources to change as well as inspectors' reports. This requires a developmental rather than a judgmental approach. Unfortunately, this is outside of the remit of HMIP.

Inspection must really be part of a package of support. First, because it could be argued that there is a duty to support change where problems are identified. Second, without support for change, inspections could paradoxically reduce the quality of service by diverting staff from their care and custodial duties.

Further, many managers already know the problems described in reports, but feel solutions are beyond their control. Limited resources and systemic obstacles prevent change, and a culture of learned helplessness soon develops. Overcrowding, now at record levels, exacerbates this. Staff are now faced with a near impossible task of maintaining standards as population levels rise and the potential for catastrophe builds.

Thus despite the presence of standards and an independent inspectorate there remains a need to support change, promote humane values and outwardly account for standards of care.

There are various ways to address this problem. First, new policy could be produced, but staff are policy-weary and policy is rarely well implemented. Education and training would probably have a little impact, but would not be sufficient. Inspection can help, but as well as the problems above, there is a fundamental problem of culture in that measurement for inspection encourages people to hide their mistakes rather than learn from them (Berwick, 1998). Something radical is needed. We propose that more prisons are run as 'therapeutic communities' (TCs) and that these are supported by a standards-based audit system embedded within a peer-support network.

Therapeutic communities and effectiveness

There are 15 democratic prison TCs in the UK – of these two are assessment units and one is for women. Only Grendon runs entirely as a TC prison. Dovegate operates within the perimeter of a larger 'main' prison while the remainder are wings in conventional prisons.

Democratic prison TCs primarily address offending behaviour and are the main focus of this chapter. There are also 'concept-based' TCs which help prisoners with addictions. These use a different model of care, albeit derived from the same root.

Therapeutic communities developed from the Northfield experiments in the 1940s (Harrison, 2000) where British Army psychiatrists attempted to rehabilitate psychologically traumatised soldiers. They focused on the group as both the patient and the intervention and aimed to stimulate learning through discussion of psychological problems and interpersonal relationships – a 'living–learning experience'. Gradually more services used this approach. In the 1960s, Rapoport described four principles that defined a therapeutic community: democracy, reality confrontation, permissiveness and communality (Rapoport, 1959). Since then these have been developed and extended and a summary of principles and their therapeutic rationale is given in Table 14.1. In 1962 HMP Grendon Underwood was established as the first democratic TC prison (Genders and Player, 1995; Morris, 2004).

Definition: *A therapeutic community is a planned environment which exploits the therapeutic value of social and group processes. It promotes equitable and democratic group-living in a varied, permissive but safe environment. Interpersonal and emotional issues are openly discussed and members can form intimate relationships. Mutual feedback helps members confront their problems and develop an awareness of interpersonal actions.*

In prisons, people volunteer to join the programme and are recruited from the general prison population. Prisoners may leave when they choose or may be voted out by the group, e.g. if they break important rules. Typically, TCs have daily community meetings, and work in large and small groups.

TCs are clinically effective. A meta-analysis conducted after a systematic review of the literature found that TCs are effective for people with personality disorders and mentally disordered offenders (Lees *et al.*, 1999). A recent study found that TCs were more effective than conventional community-based psychiatry (Chiesa *et al.*, 2004). TCs are also cost-effective (*see* chapter 16). The provision of TC care in the community can avoid the considerable cost of inappropriate use of psychiatric and prison services (Dolan *et al.*, 1996); Davies *et al.*, 1999) as described by Fiona Warren (*see* Chapter 16).

Therapeutic community prisons are proven effective even for serious offenders (Marshall, 1999; Taylor, 2000). Prison TCs have been recommended by inspectors (Ramsbotham, 2003; and *see* Chapter 15).

The Community of Communities

The Community of Communities was established in 2002 by the Royal College of Psychiatrists and the Association of Therapeutic Communities. It

Table 14.1 TC principles and therapeutic rationale

Principles	Therapeutic value or rationale
1 Democratic, participative	Allows healthy parts of the personality to emerge and be used (e.g. self-management and altruism)
2 Permissive, tolerant	Allows difficult behaviour to occur. Encourages catharsis, self-disclosure and the assumption of individual and collective responsibility.
3 Safe, boundaries	Psychological containment can be experienced and internalised.
4 Communicative, open and frank discussion	Facilitates expression of distress and understanding of its causes
5 Facilitate reality confrontation.	The consequences of actions made clear to individuals and the group.
6 Intimate, informal	Allows trust to develop, and encourages therapeutic playfulness.
7 Equitable, non-hierarchical	Demonstrates that all members are valued equally.
8 Varied environment	Allows interaction in different settings, and mutual examination of various facets of the personality
9 Communalism, group living	Helps client members explore all their interactions and provide opportunities for experimentation with new behaviours in real situations.

is a quality network of therapeutic communities that has members in the UK and abroad in health, social care, prison and special education settings. It applies a clinical audit model within a peer-support network and this fits broadly within the action–research paradigm.

Standards are the foundation of the developmental review process and are used to systematically identify areas for improvement. Each year members attend a workshop where they revise standards through discussion informed by a recent review of the literature. These include minimum standards and aspirational standards. These are applied first in self-review where staff and client members rate themselves against the standards ('met', 'partly met', 'not met') and make notes about context and reasons for non-compliance. About six weeks later the community receives a one-day visit from staff and clients from another participating community. The visitors explore problems identified in the self-review and offer advice and support. The host community, in turn, visits another community as a peer-review team.

Members receive a local report which summarises compliance with standards, areas of achievement and areas for improvement. It also notes any progress made following recommendations of the previous year's report. Later, a national report is produced which identifies trends in increased compliance and provides group means. Services can therefore compare themselves against a standard, against their previous year's performance, and against the performance of other services (benchmarking).

Finally, there is an annual members' forum. This is a chance to reflect on the process, discuss ideas for improving the process and to vote on important matters.

The network's methods and values attempt to mirror those of therapeutic communities. Central is the belief that responsibility is best promoted through interdependence. The advisory group plays a critical role in safeguarding principles, watching the burden of review and ensuring representative consultation.

Standards should reflect the underlying TC and other humane values (*see* Table 14.2) in key topic areas, ideally describing measurable attributes and behaviours. The topic areas of the standards are described in Box 14.1 and an example of a standard is given in Box 14.2. Each standard is accompanied by criteria which further describe the standard as measurable activities.

Table 14.2 Suggested humane values

---

1. Humanity
    i. Avoiding discrimination on the grounds of race, colour, religion, sex or sexual orientation
    ii. Avoiding cruel, inhuman or degrading treatment or punishment, including torture

2. Decency and dignity
    i. Avoiding abusive language
    ii. Avoiding humiliation, exploitation, coercion, oppression
    iii. Privacy

3. Care and quality of life
    i. Clean, properly equipped and maintained facilities
    ii. Meaningful and varied routine
    iii. Access to healthcare

4. Fairness
    i. Treatment of prisoners within the law – no one should be punished outside the rules
    ii. Avoiding discriminatory practice (also above)
    iii. Fair and consistent treatment
    iv. Not preventing access to entitlements

5. Safety
    i. Protecting prisoners from others and themselves
    ii. Segregating juveniles and adults
    iii. Segregating unconvicted and convicted people

Box 14.1 Topic areas of the Community of Communities standards

1. Environment and Facilities
2. Staff Members and Training
3. Joining and Leaving the Community
4. Therapeutic Milieu and Process
5. Boundaries, Containment, Responsibilities and Rights
6. Organisation, Policy and Procedures
7. External Relations and Research

Box 14.2 An example of a Community of Communities standard

1. Standard: the community uses a structured programme for therapy

Criteria

1.1 There is a structured and bounded daily programme of group activities

1.2 There are regular community meetings attended by all available client members and staff (ideally daily)

1.3 Time each working day is spent in therapeutic groups, as well as in community meetings

1.4 There is provision for crisis meetings, with a recognised procedure for calling one, that can be used by staff or client members

---

Coyle (2003a) offers a definition of 'treatment with humanity' based on four elements: preserving human dignity, respecting individuality, supporting family life and promoting personal responsibility, along with an audit tool.

Independent review and inspection is particularly important because prisons are 'total institutions' (Goffmann, 1968). This means they have different ways of working to the outside world, different cultures and are relatively impermeable. Without such an external reference, this isolation means that they are vulnerable to regimes of inhumane practice evolving. The Community of Communities network links prison TCs with TCs from the outside world.

How does the review process contribute to a humane prison?

The Community of Communities review process attempts both to demonstrate the quality of the work that goes on in prison therapeutic communities and provide an audit process which itself embodies humane principles. In this section we provide examples of the way in which the humane principles that characterise prison therapeutic communities are applied in organisational audit of prison therapeutic communities. In this way we show how the review process contributes to the ongoing development of a humane culture.

Rapoport's four key therapeutic community principles, democratisation (Table 14.1, 1), communalism (Table 14.1, 9), permissiveness (Table 14.1, 2), and reality confrontation (Table 14.1, 5) can be understood to embody humane values (Rapoport, 1959). These intersect with, but do not exhaust, the suggested humane values (Table 14.2). In prison therapeutic communities the principle of *democratisation* is implemented by involving staff and prisoners in decision-making. The community is involved in decisions about policy, the day-to-day running of the community and risk assessment of prisoners, for example, when they wish to apply for particular jobs in the community or to go for home leave.

Members of the community discuss and debate issues and then vote on them. In this way, efforts are made to flatten the hierarchy between staff and members. Such involvement of staff and prisoners encourages healthy parts of personality to emerge, such as self-management and altruism. These examples of the ways in which democratisation is implemented reflect the humane value of locating the power for decision-making with the whole group within the limits of prison security (See Table 14.2, 2.ii, 4.ii, 4.iii)

The Community of Communities review process in turn implements the principle of democratisation in comparable ways. The process is organised, run and 'owned' by staff and clients of member therapeutic communities. Thus, for example, policy decisions and the administrative running of the project are openly debated and voted on at the annual members' forum. The standards against which each community is audited have themselves been developed via a process of open consultation with all member TCs. This consultation process is repeated annually and in this way provides member ownership of the standards.

In prison TCs, the principle of *communalism* is implemented through the fostering of a culture of open communication, shared emotional and social experience, and the right of each member to speak and be heard. The intention is to generate sufficient trust to enable members to openly explore often extremely shameful and difficult personal experiences. The destructive consequences of closed secrecy so common amongst staff and members in prison is thus challenged. This provides opportunities for experimentation with new behaviours in real situations. At the heart of this endeavour is the humane value that, whatever the horrific nature of our experiences and consequent actions, each of us has the right to be understood by peers, to be accepted by peers and to be valued enough by peers in order to be given a chance to change (See Table 14.2, 1.i, 2.i, 2.ii, 4.iii).

The Community of Communities review process implements the principle of communalism by fostering a culture in which trust and frank exchange is built between communities visiting each other as part of the review process. The intention is that enough trust is built between member communities for real shortcomings to be shared and explored rather than kept secret. This would be difficult to achieve as part of a process of inspection. In this way the intention is that communities can come to understanding their often shameful difficulties and to set to work on changing them in a comparable way to the courageous journey made by individual members of a prison TC.

In prison TCs, the principle of *permissiveness* is implemented by the encouragement of the verbal expression of feelings and experiences that many members have come to feel are unacceptable – not permitted. Verbal expressions of rage and hatred are welcomed together with practically intolerable feelings of powerlessness often rooted in hitherto unspeakable experiences of physical and sexual abuse. This encourages catharsis, self-disclosure and the assumption of individual and collective responsibility. The principle of permissiveness works in tandem with clear limits, rules and boundaries about acceptable an unacceptable behaviour and actions. It is the verbal expression of hitherto unacceptable feelings that is permitted and encouraged, not the corruption of boundaries. Indeed the respect for clear limits on behaviour in relation to community members is a prerequisite for a culture of permissiveness with respect to the expression of feelings. This culture of permissiveness fostered in prison TCs again embodies the humane value that each of us has a right to have feelings about previous violations to be heard, understood and vindicated (See Table 14.2, 4.i, 4.iii).

The Community of Communities review process implements the principle of permissiveness via the inclusion and acceptance of difference across the membership and by the open encouragement of the expression and exploration of different and often traumatic experiences within member communities.

Finally, in prison TCs, the principle of *reality confrontation* is implemented by the fostering of an open culture in which members can give each other direct feedback concerning problems and unacceptable behaviours. This is encouraged in the small therapy groups and the large community meetings. The intention is that members become aware that the way they behave affects others. When members find themselves unable to engage with such reality confrontation it may be that they are voted out of the community because their behaviour is repeatedly unacceptable. This culture of reality confrontation fostered in prison therapeutic communities embodies the humane value that each of us has a right to live safely amongst others and that unacceptable behaviour will be challenged (See Table 14.2, 5.i). The Community of Communities review process implements the principle of reality confrontation via its central tenet that peer communities will scrutinise each others' practice and that consensually unacceptable practice will not be tolerated. Thus, the Community of Communities' review process mirrors therapeutic community principles which in turn reflect many of the characteristics of a humane prison.

Audit and accreditation of democratic therapeutic communities in prisons

In 1999 Her Majesty's Prison Service funded the Association of Therapeutic Communities (ATC) to develop an accreditation system for democratic TCs in prisons. The resulting Kennard and Lees Audit Checklist (KLAC) (Kennard and Lees, 2001), a list of standards based on TC values, was used as part of an annual audit.

The KLAC later informed the development of a core model for prison TCs which, like other prison programmes, is accredited by the Correctional

Services Advisory Panel. This was used for audit and replaced the KLAC. The key topic areas are described in Box 14.3 and an example of a standard is given in Box 14.4.

Box 14.3 Topic areas of the core model used to accredit democratic therapeutic communities in UK prisons

1. Institutional Support
2. Treatment and Management/Integrity
3. Continuity and Resettlement
4. Quality of Delivery

Box 14.4 Examples of standards used to audit the core model for prison TCs

1. A psychometric test battery, in accordance with the Assessment Manual (Annex 12) will be administered on completion of Therapy to inform the End of Therapy Report and Case Conference and for evaluation purposes.
2. Prisoners who are transferred from the TC at the end of treatment and remain in the prison system should be followed up by Head of Resettlement or designated manager 12 months after completing their course of treatment. There should be a tracking system in place, which includes a reminder system to ensure non/poor responses are followed up.
3. Progress in therapy is marked by a discernible qualitative difference in insight and understanding of offending between those just arrived and those who have been in treatment for a period.
4. The staff group can give clear accounts of specific criminogenic factors being addressed in therapy.

At this stage some prison TCs were participating in both Prison Service and Community of Communities audits and there was a degree of repetition in these. Consequently a new joint process was developed.

This attempts to be both a judgmental and developmental process. It is judgmental in that it provides information for the accreditation of prison TCs. Their funding is dependent on their attaining at least 60 per cent compliance with standards in certain sections. Accreditation requires stronger evidence than the developmental part of the review and so information is likely to come from several information sources and is more rigorously checked.

Key stages of the joint review process

The joint review process uses a two-day visit. Day 1 is a supportive Community of Communities peer-review day. On Day 2, a psychologist, prison service representative and TC expert observe the therapeutic programme in action and collect the data to audit the TC against the accredited model. The psychologist conducts two case studies to provide detailed information about how the programme addresses offending behaviour. Prisoners' records are audited and information about standards critical for accreditation is collected. Feedback is given at the end of both days and later in a more detailed local report. A national report provides a detailed comparison of all prison TCs' performance.

Limitations of standards

Audit is a confirmatory approach as it is concerned with the extent to which standards have been met. Unfortunately, this means that it is limited in its ability to detect and evaluate innovative practice not described by the standards. This may result in a drive towards uniformity that stifles innovation and creativity. In addition, measuring compliance does not explain problems or how improvements could be made. For this reason the Community of Communities method includes exploratory questions in its data collection tools.

Many organisational standards describe processes rather than outcomes. It could therefore be argued that they dictate how things should be done, rather than what is achieved, and hence are over-prescriptive and miss the point. The standards' rationale is not often given although it is usually clear that they contribute in some way to better outcomes, such as reduced recidivism or service cost. Any improvements in outcomes would probably be very small at first and as outcome measurement is crude this would be hard to detect. The Community of Communities network would ideally incorporate or link into a system of routine outcomes measurement.

The relationship between staff and prisoners is critical and has the greatest influence on whether the prison has a human or an inhuman environment (Coyle, 2003b). It is important that standards are measurable, but the staff–prisoner relationship is hard to measure and hence is not well covered by the standards. This means that a prison with very poor staff–prisoner relationships (e.g. mistrust, violence, antagonism), could 'tick all the boxes' but fail to deliver a good service. The challenge then is to: (i) identify standards that are critical to care provided; (ii) resist removing these standards from data collection tools on the grounds that they are hard to measure; and (iii) identify reliable methods to collect information about these.

The process of developing standards should be empowering. The standards will communicate group consensus on best practice. They also help define members' responsibilities, and the process of involving front-line staff and members has an educational and training function which should not be underestimated.

Standards help clarify goals and values and give us a vision of something better. This is fundamental to the success of any organisational change process. Discussing the standards can also help people question the status quo and realise that it is within the power of the group to make radical changes if necessary. This would need to include the senior management team. While the idea of radical change can be daunting, discussing standards and better ways of working often serves as an impetus for small experiments and thus incremental change. Regular attainment of achievable targets sustains motivation.

Limitations of the method

Frank discussion is likely to be limited in the new joint review process by the fact that accreditation is part of the joint visit. It will be harder for staff and prisoners to trust their peer-reviewers knowing they must soon show their best for the purposes of accreditation. The problem is that measurement for inspection encourages people to hide their errors instead of learn from them (Berwick, 1998).

The process is also very limited by the short time available on site and the amount of standards that must be checked in that time. A report from the Cabinet Office's Public Sector Team recognised the serious opportunity costs of preparing for inspection meant staff were being diverted from the task of healthcare delivery (Cabinet Office, 2003).

Those prison therapeutic communities most in need of support may paradoxically be those least able to engage in the process. There is a considerable amount of time required to involve staff and members in the self-review, in preparing for the peer-review and to follow up action plans systematically. Senior managers should be aware that this can be a burden on staff teams, and extra support should be provided, particularly to teams with depleted numbers, during busy times of the review process

Some staff have commented that an annual cycle gives too little time to implement change between reviews.

Pros, cons and critical questions

In this section we provide a summary box of the pros and cons of the standards-based peer-review model and quality improvement (*see* Box 14.5). We also highlight questions for policy makers and senior managers. It is critical that these questions are addressed if the development of quality improvement and monitoring of standards within the Prison Service is to be underpinned by humane values in the way that we have argued it should be (see questions 1, 2 and 3). In addition, we highlight questions concerning how best to implement the process of peer-review based on humane values in the context of prisons (see question 4).

Box 14.5 Pros and cons of standards-based peer-review

Pros
1. Helps clarify goals and values
2. Systematic way to identify areas for improvement and areas of achievement
3. Enables and empowers staff and prisoners; networks can also lobby senior figures on their behalf

4. Standards represent consensus
5. Safeguards and promotes values
6. Low cost
7. Allows incremental improvement
8. Educative – staff learn about standards
9. Represents service development needs to senior managers and funders
10. Networking helps reduce isolation
11. Promotes learning – members share info and process encourage open and honest reflection

Cons
1. Adds to the bureaucratic burden of regulation and review
2. Creates a culture of mistrust of professionals – could rely on professionals' reflective practice and years of training and experience
3. A defence against anxiety
4. Oversimplistic as critical parts of the service are missed because they are hard to measure, e.g. prison culture, staff morale, trust between therapist and inmate
5. Accreditation is judgmental and thus inherently unsupportive
6. It creates a culture of fear and blame and encourages lying not learning
7. May encourage uniformity and stifle innovation
8. Over-zealous inspectors versus genuine peers

1 **Efficiency: a programme of support versus behaviourist intervention?**
The new policy of standards and target-setting and inspectorate and performance monitoring, is essentially a structural approach to reform. It views organisations as structures of discrete components performing discrete tasks rather than systems with interacting subcomponents and in an external context. Furthermore, systems of 'earned autonomy', for example, as described in the NHS Plan (Department of Health, 2000), allow better performing services to manage their own affairs and choose how they spend funds whereas poorer performers have these decisions made for them. Coercive approaches use specific pressure and control, including legislation, litigation, licensing, accreditation and budgeting. Failing services may even have their management franchised to private companies. This kind of 'organisational behaviour modification' is based on classical theories of conditioning and controlling behaviour and there are similarities with behaviourism and associated techniques such as positive and negative reinforcement. We suggest that it is paramount to explore the question of whether it is more efficient to offer a programme of support such as the democratic peer-review process as described in this chapter rather than just simple reward and punishment.

2 **Peer-review and accreditation: an irreconcilable tension?**
The joint review process described in this chapter carries with it an

inherent tension rooted in the different aspirations of the developmental and judgmental components intrinsic in the Community of Communities and Prison Service Accreditation Audit respectively. The question of whether the prison therapeutic community remains an accredited programme hangs on the audit. This has implications not only for the performance targets of the organisation at senior management level but also for the targets of front-line staff. Such a process can encourage staff at all levels to hide weaknesses in their service and hence not learn from them. The Community of Communities peer-review process by contrast is not driven by the task of accreditation, but rather an aim is to encourage open discussion to enable learning. There is a danger that the humane values embedded in the Community of Communities peer-review process (as a reflection of therapeutic community values), might be drowned by the efforts of staff to demonstrate that they meet their management targets. While efforts are being made to address this tension, an important question remains as to whether this will be resolved in the coming years.

3 **Clinical governance and the burdens of inspection: lessons to learn from the NHS?**
Clinical governance is now becoming increasingly well embedded in the management structure and strategies within the NHS and has particular relevance for ensuring and monitoring quality as well as implementing service improvements. Within the context of the aspiration for humane prisons it seems highly relevant to ask: Could a clinical governance framework help prison services? We suggest it will be critical to explore and address the questions of what such a clinical governance framework might look like and how it might be implemented within the prison service with particular reference to the experiences of staff and patients across the organisation in the NHS.

The important issue of whether inspection and monitoring per se provide a real chance for reform or just simply more bureaucracy is addressed with respect to the NHS in the report of the Cabinet Office Public Sector Team and the Department of Health (Cabinet Office, 2003). Drawing on the lessons learnt in the NHS, we suggest it is now critical in the context of the prison service to explore and address the following questions: What are the burdens of inspection and monitoring? How can it go right? How can it all go wrong?

4 **Involving all members of the Prison, including the 'service user', in a peer-review process: can it be done?**
As has been highlighted, a central feature of the democratic and thus humane nature of the prison service and Community of Communities joint review process is the active encouragement of member involvement in the audit cycle. Such involvement is partially built into the process insofar as member views are sought in the self-review workbook prior to the peer visit. Additionally, meetings are automatically timetabled to gather the views of members during the peer-review visits. Further, the project actively encourages members to be active in the visiting peer-review teams alongside staff.

In some participating TCs, members have also been involved in other aspects of the annual peer-review cycle. Thus in some communities a 'Community of Communities' working group has been set up. Membership of such a working group has generally consisted of a mix of representative staff and members. The group has usually been tasked by the wider community to take a lead on ensuring the self-review workbook is completed in a way that represents all members' views. Additionally, they have been given responsibility for ensuring that every member of the community is aware of what the peer-review is, of the peer-review timetable, of who the peer-review visitors will be, of why they will be there and of what they will be interested in exploring. The working group has encouraged members to use the peer-review experience to speak as openly and frankly as they wish about anything they wish. In this way, such examples of Community of Communities working groups have managed to go as far as they can to ensure that all members are prepared emotionally and practically for the audit and can subsequently participate in it in an informed way.

Following the peer-review visit, once the peer-review report has been prepared, such working groups have been tasked to take a lead on communicating to the wider community areas that were considered to be an achievement. They have been given responsibility for making action plans for ensuring that areas identified for improvement are addressed where it is in the community's power to effect change. Such involvement of members in the preparation for and follow up of the peer-review visits has been intended to foster a culture in which members of the prison therapeutic communities feel empowered to take part in improving the quality of their community.

In practice, this ideal aim of empowerment of front-line staff and members has usually been achieved in part only, for front-line staff and members have the power to change a limited number of things, such as the quality of training and clinical supervision (front-line staff) or the quality and quantity of activities done informally with staff and members together (front-line staff and members). Many of the areas of improvement in the action plans lie beyond the remit of frontline staff as they concern issues at the organisational level (usually involving cost) for which senior managers have responsibility. For example, it is often in the hands of the senior managers as to how consistently staff are deployed, whether financial resources are given to providing more telephones, soundproofing between therapy rooms, larger dining rooms to enable all staff and members to eat together, and so forth. In practice, when senior managers find themselves having to make difficult decisions about how to spend restricted financial resources, such areas for improvement that lie in their domain may understandably go unattended to. When the same areas for improvement are fed back to a therapeutic community each year, this can have the effect of creating scepticism and disillusionment in the front-line staff and members of the prison TCs about the worth of the review process. We suggest that this underlines the central importance of the question of how to ensure the full support and involvement of senior managers in the review process.

Conclusion

Many UK prisons do not provide humane care or conditions. The government must address overcrowding by either reducing prison sentencing or building more prisons. It must also provide proper mental healthcare. But this is not sufficient. A peer-review process, such as the one described in this chapter, can help safeguard and promote humane prisons if it is based on standards that are grounded in humane values.

Acknowledgments

Prison TC members who have participated in the Community of Communities, the Community of Communities project team, Sunita Patel and Gina Pearce, Andrew Edwards and Paul Lelliott.

References

Berwick D (1998) The NHS: feeling well and thriving at 75. *BMJ*. **317**: 57–61.

Cabinet Office Public Sector Team and the Department of Health (2003) *Making a Difference: Reducing burdens in healthcare inspection and monitoring*. Cabinet Office, London.

Chiesa M, Fonagy P, Holmes J et al. (2004) Residential versus community treatment of personality disorder: A comparative study of three treatments. *American Journal of Psychiatry*. **161**: 1463–70.

Coyle A (2002) *Managing Prisons in a Time of Change*. International Centre for Prison Studies, London.

Coyle A (2003a) *A Human Rights Approach to Prison Management*. International Centre for Prison Studies, London.

Coyle A (2003b) *Humanity in Prison: questions of definition and audit*. International Centre for Prison Studies, London.

Davies S (1999) Does every district need a therapeutic community? In: P Campling and R Haigh (eds) *Therapeutic Communities: past, present and future*. Jessica Kingsley, London.

Dodd V (2003) Brutality of prison officers exposed. *The Guardian*. **11 December**. www.guardian.co.uk/prisons/story/0,,1104506,00.html.

Department of Health (2000) *The NHS Plan: A plan for investment, a plan for reform*. Crown copyright.

Department of Health (1997) *The New NHS: modern, dependable*. HMSO, London.

Dolan BM, Warren F, et al. (1996) Cost-offset following specialist treatment of severe personality disorders. *Psychiatric Bulletin*. **20**: 413–17.

Genders E and Player E (1995) *Grendon: A Study of a Therapeutic Prison*. Oxford University Press, Oxford.

Goffman E (1968) *Asylums: essays on the social situation of mental patients and other inmates*. Penguin, Harmondsworth.

Harrison T (2000) Bion, Rickman, Foulkes and the Northfield Experiments. Jessica Kingsley, London.

Her Majesty's Inspectorate of Prisons (2005) *Annual Report of HM Chief Inspector of Prisons for England and wales 2003-2004*. The Stationery Office, London.

Her Majesty's Inspectorate of Prisons (2004) *Expectations: criteria for assessing the conditions in prisons and the treatment of prisoners* (2e). HMIP, London. See: http://inspectorates.homeoffice.gov.uk/hmiprisons/docs/expectations.pdf.

Her Majesty's Inspectorate of Prisons (2005) *Report on a full announced inspection of HM/YOI Feltham, 15–20 May 2005.* HMIP, London.

International Centre for Prison Studies (2004) *Humanising the Treatment of Prisoners.* Guidance Note 9. International Centre for Prison Studies, London.

Joint Committee On Human Rights (2004) *Third Report.* House of Lords and the House of Commons, London.

Kennard D and Lees K (2001) *Kennard Lees Audit Checklist 2.* www.therapeutic communities.org/klac.htm.

Lees J, Manning N and Rawlings B (1999) *CRD Report 17 – Therapeutic Community Effectiveness: a systematic international review of therapeutic community treatment for people with personality disorders and mentally disordered offenders.* Centre for Reviews and Dissemination, University of York, York.

Marshall P (1999) *A Reconviction Study of HMP Grendon.* Research Findings 53. www.homeoffice.gov.uk/rds/pdfs/r53.pdf.

Morgan R (2002) Imprisonment. In: M Maguire, R Morgan, R Reiner (eds) *The Oxford Handbook of Criminology* (3e). Oxford University Press, Oxford

Morris M (2004) *Dangerous and Severe: process, programme and person: Grendon's work.* Jessica Kingsley, London.

Office for National Statistics (1998) *Psychiatric Morbidity among Prisoners in England and Wales.* Department of Health, London. www.statistics.gov.uk/downloads/theme_health/Prisoners_PsycMorb.pdf.

Ramsbotham D (2003) *Prisongate: the shocking state of Britain's prisons and the need for visionary change.* Free Press, London.

Rapoport, RN (1959) *Community as Doctor.* Tavistock, London.

Royal College of Psychiatrists (2002) *Suicide in Prisons.* Royal College of Psychiatrists, London.

Taylor R (2000) *A Seven-year Reconviction Study of HMP Grendon Therapeutic Community.* Research Findings No. 115. Home Office, London. Available at: www.homeoffice.gov.uk/rds/pdfs/r115.pdf.

Travis A (2001) Jails chief threatens to resign. *The Guardian.* **6 February**. http://society.guardian.co.uk/crimeandpunishment/story/0,,434177,00.html.

Wilson D (2005) *Death at the Hands of the State.* Howard League for Penal Reform, London.

Chapter 15

Independent inspection of prisons

Anne Owers, Her Majesty's Chief Inspector of Prisons

> The objective of the present Protocol is to establish a system of regular visits undertaken by independent international and national bodies to places where people are deprived of their liberty, in order to prevent torture and other cruel, inhuman or degrading treatment or punishment.
>
> > Optional Protocol to the UN Convention against torture and other cruel, inhuman or degrading treatment or punishment, December 2003

> Inspector to prison chaplain: Do you know what the Inspectorate is?
> Chaplain (smiling): Oh, yes. You're the people who make potted plants appear.
> > Conversation during inspection of private prison, 2003

Those are the extremes of prison inspection. At the highest level, the independent monitoring of places of custody is mandated under international law, as an essential safeguard for the human rights and proper treatment of those the state holds in custody. It can point up or seek to prevent abuse, or signal the need for fundamental systemic change. But prisons are total institutions; and at a much more mundane level, inspection can serve to ameliorate some of the dehumanising effects of imprisonment on lives whose every movement and choice is controlled: access to clean and decent clothing, showers, phones – and even greenery.

The prisons inspectorate of England and Wales has existed, in its present form, since 1981. Its statutory remit is to report, to the Home Secretary, on conditions in prisons and the treatment of prisoners, since extended to include conditions and treatment in immigration removal (i.e. detention) centres. Unlike other inspectorates, it does not inspect or report on a service, its cost-effectiveness or efficiency: it reports on an institution, its culture, decency and safety. Nor is it bound by the standards that the institution, whether publicly or privately run, is contracted to deliver. It inspects by its own criteria, referenced to international human rights standards, which define what constitutes a 'healthy' prison or custodial environment.

A healthy prison appears even more of an oxymoron than a humane prison. Prison, by definition, is unnatural, stressful and restrictive. Nevertheless, within those limits, our inspectorate looks for environments that can satisfy four key tests: that prisoners, even the most vulnerable, are held safely; that they are treated with respect for their human dignity, whatever their offence; that they are engaged in activity which has a purpose and which is likely to enhance their skills; and that they are prepared for return to the community, however far off that may be.

Each of those tests is assessed by examining in detail all the aspects of prison life, from first reception to eventual discharge: taking in healthcare, education and training, use of force and segregation, experiences of bullying or self-harm, relationships with other prisoners and staff. Our detailed criteria, which we call *Expectations*, are based not upon minimum auditable standards, but best practice. They do not examine whether targets are met – targets often measure what is measurable, not what is important. Our criteria test quality, not compliance. They may point to a systemic failure, that stretches across, and even beyond, the Prison Service. They do not, as such, look at value for money – what price a suicide? – though they may well reveal that resources are wasted, or staff or managers insufficiently active. They are referenced against international human rights standards and have now been exported to other countries. They have been welcomed by the Foreign Office's human rights department, have been used to inspect women's prisons in Canada, and, on a recent trip to the US, were avidly seized on by non-governmental organisations and prisons administrators keen to reform and develop a system of monitoring for US prisons.

Before all full inspections, researchers carry out confidential random surveys of prisoners, to discern their experience of all aspects of imprisonment. The results of those surveys can be compared against other similar prisons, or against the same prison at its last inspection. During inspections, inspectors have full access (with their own keys) to all parts of the prison, its documents and its staff. They will observe, read, talk and listen for a full week. The seven-strong multidisciplinary team includes those with operational prisons experience, but also those from social work, probation and other backgrounds. It will include a healthcare specialist and a drugs specialist, and the team will work alongside a parallel team of education inspectors, who will examine the provision of education and training.

The outcome of the inspection will be a detailed report, with recommendations for improvement. All inspection reports are published, in the form and at the time that the Chief Inspector decides; and prisons must then produce an action plan, which a subsequent inspection will check. Though our recommendations are not mandatory, around 92 per cent are accepted, and we find on reinspection that over 70 per cent have been achieved, wholly or partially, within about two years.

At least half of our inspections take place without any warning, so that the potted plants have no chance to be ordered, corridors painted, staff primed or the segregation unit emptied. This is one of the most important weapons in our armoury. Our inspectors have a lot of territory to cover: 138 prisons, holding a record number of prisoners (over 77 500 in October 2005). Each prison will be visited at least twice in a five-year period: once for a full inspection and again to check whether the recommendations of that inspection have been actioned. It is not enough. But our right to turn up anywhere at any time means that every prison governor in the country knows we can knock on his prison gate today. That knowledge is a kind of virtual inspection; and we have developed an intelligence system that alerts us to those places where the virtual needs to become real. Those prisons will see us more often, and usually without warning.

Independent Monitoring Boards: bringing the outside in

We are also only one part of the whole system for monitoring prisons and places of detention. Each prison has an Independent Monitoring Board (IMB), a group of unpaid local people with statutory authority to go into that prison, receive requests and complaints from prisoners, monitor the use of segregation, and report any concerns to the governor. In addition, the Prisons and Probation Ombudsman (PPO) can investigate individual complaints from prisoners which have not been satisfactorily resolved in the internal complaints procedures, and, as of last year, must carry out investigations into all deaths in custody, whether natural, self-inflicted or homicide.

This provides a complementary system of independent oversight, of which independent inspection is a crucial part. IMBs are there all the time but need to maintain a relationship with their prison, and may not be aware of its idiosyncrasies. The PPO can address individual complaints, but may not see the broader picture. Inspection provides a holistic view of each prison or place of detention, carried out by independent experts, which can compare one prison to others and can also set all prisons against independent human rights-based criteria.

What, then, are the achievements of, and the barriers to, independent inspection? Prisons are closed environments, which can easily become self-referential, and where the obvious need for security can easily become an end in itself or an excuse for poor practice or unnecessary control. Prison reform is most likely to happen when an outside eye is applied to what goes on, and when outside observers ask why it is so.

Most recent developments in prisons in England and Wales have happened as a result of bringing the outside in: of applying to services provided in prisons the norms and expectations that would apply were those services delivered in the community. Prison healthcare, for example, was notoriously poor and this was highlighted in an inspectorate thematic report in 1997. Sometimes it was staffed by people who would never have been allowed to practise outside prison; nowhere was it subject to stringent standards of clinical governance. Since then, it has undergone a sea-change, with the aim of making the service provided in prisons equivalent to that provided outside, to the extent that prison healthcare is now commissioned, and paid for, by the same Primary Care Trusts that provide healthcare for the rest of the community and must operate to the same standards.

Similarly, education and training in prisons was something marginal: its budget liable to be raided by a needy governor and its provision patchy (and access to it unreliable). That, too, has improved considerably: with ringfenced budgets provided by the Department for Education and Skills, provision delegated to local Learning and Skills Councils, and an inspection regime that uses the same standards as those applied to schools or further education colleges in the community. There is still not enough education and training of the right kind: in our last annual report, we found that only 5 of the 18 training prisons we inspected had enough education and training. There are still too many prisons where it is not seen as core to the prison's role, and where staff may make prisoners' attendance difficult, or certainly not encourage it. In one recent inspection, staff coming on duty cheered when the tannoy system announced that education had been cancelled that day. And its provision is too often mechanistic: a 'one size fits all' approach that does not recognise and seek to meet prisoners' individual needs, in particular the fact that, having avoided or been avoided by education all their lives, they may need to approach it by a side wind, acquiring literacy and numeracy in order to carry out other tasks – whether that is car mechanics or pottery. But it is nevertheless a greatly improved picture.

Resettlement, too, has become part of the active vocabulary of prisons over the last four or five years. The question of what comes next, the need to marry up any positive work done in prisons with support and interventions after release, has not only led to more joined-up work in many individual prisons, but also to an attempted restructuring of the whole prison and probation services into a unified National Offender Management Service. The aims of these changes are positive – to construct an end-to-end system around the needs of each individual offender. But their effective implementation is problematic, hampered by the scale of the task in a prison system that has no headroom and no additional resources available to carry it out. People who end up in prison have often never been 'settled': they will face multiple problems on release. There are no quick fixes, yet there is a danger that politicians will expect immediate and unachievable results.

These are some of the gains that have been stimulated and encouraged by regular inspection. Crucially, they have involved seeing prisoners as people (patients, learners, workers), not simply as offenders. This can have a significant impact on a custodial environment – not just the direct benefits it can provide for prisoners, but the signal to all those working there that their task is not simply containment, or even 'treatment', but normalisation.

Overcrowding

However, there are huge barriers in the way of making further improvements and even sustaining those that have been made. The main barrier is overcrowding, and this is now built into the system. Our prisons are 24 per cent overcrowded and are expected to operate at this level.

Overcrowding is corrosive. Overcrowded prisons are places where two prisoners routinely share a cell meant for one where they eat all their meals, sometimes in the presence of an unscreened toilet. They may spend 23 hours a day there. Living in a lavatory in any other public building would contravene any number of public health and decency standards, yet it is an accepted part of prison life. Alternatively, prisoners may lack in-cell sanitation at all and be dependent upon a call-bell system, where a combination of unreliable systems, less than assiduous staff, security considerations and over-demand can mean that they 'slop out' – sometimes, as we reported at Portland Young Offenders Institution, out of the window, sometimes, as in women's prisons, when pregnant or menstruating. Further, as at Norwich or Leeds, they may be held in wings that are unfit for habitation. The Prison Service has no wish to hold prisoners in those conditions. But it has no space, or resources, to close down, or reconfigure, those establishments, as this would reduce the number of prison places.

Self-harm, suicide and the duty of care

Population pressure also undermines prisons' ability to exercise their duty of care, the duty to preserve life. The rate of all deaths in custody is increasing: but the rate of self-inflicted deaths has reached a new high of around two deaths a week, though overall numbers have declined somewhat during the last year. Self-inflicted deaths have become part of the currency of penal life: in a recent week where there were six, this did not even make the news. Most of those who kill themselves in our prisons are among the most vulnerable of prisoners: new to custody, sometimes not even sentenced, often detoxifying from drugs, mentally ill, in prison healthcare or segregation. The connection between overcrowding and suicide is clear. Earlier this year, the prison population stabilised: so did the suicide rate. From April to August, the population shot up to a new high of over 77 000: at the same time, there were 39 suicides in prisons, nearly all in the local prisons that receive large numbers of prisoners, fresh to prison, when they are most vulnerable and their risks and needs least known. But during this period, the women's prison population remained at lower levels than before, giving prisons precious space to try to manage and support some very damaged women: and the suicide rate among women also dipped.

The Prison Service has undoubtedly made considerable efforts to prevent and reduce suicide and self-harm in prison, spurred on in part by an inspectorate thematic report on suicides in prison. Systems, procedures and guidance for managing those at risk of suicide or self-harm have been developed. And the pattern of self-injury is now monitored.

Part of the role of an inspectorate is to check that those procedures are applied rigorously. But our role is also to point to the underlying causes of the epidemic of suicide and self-harm: the vulnerability of those entering prison, and the additional vulnerability that results from incarceration. Recent studies have shown that suicide rates in prison do not necessarily correlate with vigilance in carrying out protective procedures (Shaw, 2003). Organisations are good at process, at designing procedures. But suicide prevention is about something much more subtle and important. Suicide rates correlate very strongly with prisoners' feelings of distress, principally whether they feel safe, and this in turn depends upon right and respectful relationships with staff, other prisoners and their families. So, the human dignity that is at the heart of human rights compliance is also at the heart of suicide prevention.

Inspections can capture that quality of life better than standards and targets can: by observing what is going on, talking to staff and prisoners, and carrying out confidential prisoner surveys. They can detect the difference between two prisons, similar in function, resources and population: where one is perceptibly safe and decent, in spite of low staff numbers and prisoners being out of their cells most of the day, and the other is edgy, unkempt and with a drug subculture.

However, there are important protective measures that prisons must take in respect of their duty of care to those they hold. Prisoners are particularly vulnerable in the early days in custody, not least because many are withdrawing from drugs. In a 2002 report on Styal women's prison, we found women 'fitting and vomiting' in their cells for want of adequate detoxification. We called for urgent action. Eighteen months later, a proper detoxification regime was put in place – too late for the six women who had died in the intervening period, all in the early days of custody, all with a serious drug habit. And the absence of proper detoxification at Styal was not for want of knowing what it was, or how it should be delivered. The women's policy group in the prison service had developed effective treatment for drug withdrawal, specific to the substance use problems of women. But no one ensured that it was put in place, as a matter of urgency, in a prison where around 70% of women were withdrawing from drugs. It was not because staff did not care (they did) but they were engaged in crisis management, in a prison that was barely coping with the scale of demand it faced – engaged in fire-fighting rather than planned prevention. It is welcome that there have been no deaths at Styal in the two years since proper detoxification was put in place, and that detoxification generally, particularly in the women's estate, has improved considerably. That has undoubtedly been spurred on, and resources levered out of the system, because of the combined pressure of case law, inquiries and inspection.

A raft of new processes and procedures for investigating deaths in custody is now being put in place, inspired by the Article 2 obligations now imported into English law via the Human Rights Act. *Middleton* and *Creamer* have established coroners' duty to inquire into the circumstances, as well as the causes, of death (House of Lords, 2004, Para. 27), hopefully in the context of a complete review of coronial powers and procedures. And inquests, increasingly, are recording verdicts of systemic failure. The Prison and Probation Ombudsman is now charged with investigating all deaths in custody and in probation hostels. Mounting speedy investigations and producing swift conclusions that can seek to prevent recurrence will be a challenge. But these inquiries and inquests are only part of the picture. Inevitably, they start from the inability of the state to keep alive someone in its care. In our view, inquiries should also follow near-death incidents, both because the Article 2 arguments are equally strong, and because the reasons and circumstances can better be established and preventive measures taken. And inspection, equally, is an important part of prevention.

Population pressure and shared cells have implications for prisoners' safety, as well as human dignity. Those shared cells are inhabited by a transitory population, often arriving late and in numbers from court, or being moved around from prison to prison to make space for the next new arrivals. When the pressure is at its highest, prisons and the prison service are effectively playing a gruesome game of musical cells. Though the pressure has reduced somewhat, it is still there. The cases of Christopher Edwards (ECHR, 2002) and Zahid Mubarek (House of Lords, 2003) vividly show the risks inherent in cell sharing with others who may be violent or psychotic. Prisons need to carry out rigorous risk assessments before making those decisions. A few still do not, or do so scantily; and we point that out in inspections.

But consider what prisons are being asked to do. A prisoner arrives, perhaps with 30 or 40 others, in the late afternoon or early evening, in many cases still withdrawing from drugs. Leeds prison was settling in 438 new prisoners in a month; Pentonville was coping with 3000 prisoner movements each month. Each prisoner may carry with them only a court warrant. In a short interview, in a crowded reception area, before locking prisoners down for the night, staff must establish, largely from the prisoner him or herself, and from their own observations and experience, whether prisoners pose a risk to themselves or others – and then, juggling the few available spaces, place each one safely, either alone or with a suitable cell-mate.

Arriving at a new prison is a time of maximum vulnerability for prisoners. Yet prison staff are not helped by the fact that getting prisoners to prison at a reasonable time does not have the same priority for escort contractors, or the courts themselves, as getting them to court on time. Governors can face contempt proceedings for the latter; there are no penalties for the former, such as the mentally ill young man, with a history of self-harm and a recent family bereavement, who was sent to prison for a mental health assessment by a judge at 10.40 a.m. and did not arrive in the Young Offender Institution until 8.30 p.m. As often happens, prison reception staff stayed well beyond the end of their shift, but they were unable to deal with his considerable problems fully by that time.

Mental health and vulnerable prisoners

In my annual report of 2004, I focused on the issue of mental health in prisons. The first European Court of Human Rights' finding of an Article 3 violation in relation to UK prison conditions was in the case of *Keenan*. Mark Keenan was diagnosed with paranoid schizophrenia and personality disorder. He spent his time in prison being shuffled between the healthcare centre (where he attacked staff) and the segregation unit (where he eventually killed himself).

In the last three and a half years, I have seen many Mark Keenans, still alive. In some cases, they are awaiting transfer to an NHS secure facility. This, though quicker than it used to be, still takes up to three months, during which time significant deterioration can occur, in an environment that, despite the best efforts of staff, is not essentially therapeutic and cannot treat severe mental illness without the patient's consent. When asked how long he thought a prisoner in this condition should wait before transfer, the Head of Prison Healthcare, at a recent conference, said, 'If it were a relative of mine, no more than a day or two.'

Others, however, have been returned from secure facilities as too disruptive to manage – such as a young man of 18, in a body belt for three days, because without it he tore strips off his anti-tear clothing and tried to hang himself; if given a television, he broke the glass and ate it. Thanks to considerable and commendable efforts by the Prison Service, he was re-sectioned and re-admitted to a secure NHS hospital. When I inspected one women's prison recently, the healthcare centre had a row of stools outside three of the cells.

Outside each sat an agency nurse, literally watching the prisoner at all times. Inside each was a mentally ill young woman, including one who came to the door, begging to be let out because her voices were tormenting her, and who had already tied nine ligatures that morning. Daily in our prisons, governors try to keep such prisoners safe, while also respecting their human dignity and the safety of other prisoners and staff. And daily their vulnerability is increased by imprisonment, like the girl in one prison with Asperger's syndrome, held in a healthcare centre that mainly contained mentally ill and severely self-harming adult women: it was a feature of her condition that she mimicked the behaviour around her.

Other Mark Keenans are no longer alive. One in five of those who kill themselves in prison do so in segregation units or hospitals and most are mentally ill: indeed, in some prisons we visit, like Feltham Young Offender Institution, it is impossible to get a bed in the prison hospital if you are merely physically ill. The prison service's strategies for coping are often less than ideal, born out of desperation, not care planning. Like Mark Keenan, many prisoners are shuffled between healthcare and segregation, to offer respite for staff – or from prison to prison in a policy known as 'sale or return' where governors pass the parcel of their most difficult and disruptive prisoners. One young man who killed himself had been in 30 prisons in 18 months.

These are extreme cases: as are all potential human rights violations. But they are the tip of an iceberg of chronic mental instability and depression: some statistics put this as high as 80 per cent of the prison population. In one report, we described the 'quiet despair' of those who are not so acutely ill that they demand constant attention. It is undoubtedly the case that mental heath provision in prisons has improved and is set to improve still further. Under the new commissioning arrangements with primary care trusts, many prisons now have mental health in-reach teams; some have daycare centres. But those teams are still fire-fighting; in most cases they can only deal with those whose mental health problems are severe and enduring, rather than chronic and sporadic.

It is important to chronicle and inspect the treatment and conditions for those prisoners; and to uphold their human rights. But we also have to ask deeper questions – principally whether prison is the right place, or can ever provide the right environment, especially in overcrowded prisons where prisoners, particularly 'difficult' prisoners, may be locked up most of the day. We are using our prisons as society's 'too difficult' tray, in which to contain (and it is little more than that in many cases), usually for short but repeat periods, those for whom there is no proper provision outside prison, or who have already been excluded from society. They include the mentally ill, as well as young people who have been in care, excluded or truanted from school, those addicted to drugs and alcohol. And we are asking prisons to do this on the cheap. In a local male prison, where many of those prisoners are to be found, the average cost of a prisoner place is £30 000 a year; a bed in a regional secure NHS facility costs £136 000; for women in local prisons, the relative costs are £36 000 and £163 000. Those differences are a precise measure of the difference in the number of skilled staff available to treat and work with the patient.

Similar points can be made in relation to children. The children who end up in our prisons are the most difficult and damaged in society. They are cared for by staff who have very limited training in the care of disturbed adolescents, at a fraction of the cost of a local authority secure home, and outside the direct scope of the Children Act. Resources and facilities for them have considerably improved, but our inspections continue to raise concerns about some of the very vulnerable young people held in prisons. Recent cases have helped greatly in clarifying both the fact that the children themselves are within scope of the Act, and that local authorities, and particularly Area Child Protection Committees, cannot divest themselves of their responsibilities for safeguarding those children simply because they are incarcerated.

Why inspection?

Incarceration is, in this country, the most severe penalty that can be exacted: it therefore requires the most robust scrutiny. Prisons are, by definition, hidden from public view. They face some difficult human rights dilemmas, looking after people that society outside has given up on, or does not want to deal with. But they are also places that can and do become self-referential, lacking the external checks and balances that make institutions ask difficult questions, rather than revert to a default setting of institutional convenience. At their very worst, they can degrade those they hold. The pictures from Abu Ghraib in Iraq are a potent reminder of what unchecked custodial power can do. There are others. In the mid-nineteenth century, English local prisons were transformed into agents of carefully graded punishment by Edward Du Cane, using the treadmill and the crank, such that one judge considered a two year sentence in such a jail to be 'next only to death' in severity of sentence. Sean McConville (1994), in his book of that name, reminds us:

> If we define power as the enforcement of will irrespective of the wishes of the person upon whom it is enforced, the system of local imprisonment developed in England from the 1860s onwards was, above all, an exercise in power. Cut loose from the restraints of community and traditional ethical moorings, it came close to a confusion of means with ends, and a belief that any means was justified short of permanent disablement, death or the personal caprice or advantage of the captor . . . [It had] but one intent: to suppress resistance and to ensure that, whatever was going on in the mind of the offender, he would submit or be broken.

That is, thank goodness, light years away from anything I have observed in any of the custodial settings I have inspected. But it indicates the power, and the isolation, within a closed environment. And there have been abuses in our prisons within recent years. Prisons can go bad very quickly: the balance of power is always with the custodian, not the detainee.

Prison inspecting is an essential part of those 'community and traditional ethical moorings' that McConville found lacking in the late nineteenth century. Indeed, as he points out, the development of a harsh and essentially punitive system was paralleled by the emasculation of the powers of prison inspectors, some of whom had previously been robust critics of slopping out, and the use of degrading work, but who became subsumed into the work of the

Prison Commissioners, who ran prisons. At the same time, the powers of local justices of the peace (the community watchdogs, forerunners of independent monitoring boards) were also curtailed.

I have rarely been into a prison where inspection did not reveal something that those running it did not know, or had ignored. There is sometimes a 'virtual prison' – the one that exists in the governor's office, at headquarters, in the minister's red boxes – as compared with the actual prison being operated on the ground. Inspections pick up the 'inspection gaps' between what ought to be and what is. Some of them seem minor by comparison with the extreme issues I have raised earlier but they are all important to the human dignity of those held in custody.

For example, adjudication is the process by which offences against prison discipline are judged and punished. Punishments can include: cellular confinement in segregation, sometimes without access to any external stimulation except a Bible; loss of the meagre prison earnings (therefore, no tobacco, no additional food); loss of association (and therefore access to phones and contact with families). There is no independent judge, no defence lawyer to hold the ring. In one prison we inspected recently, we observed adjudications where a prisoner was cautioned, without being found guilty; where a complete defence was ignored; where no mitigation was sought; and where the only word on the adjudication sheet was 'guilty'. In another prison, a woman who had tried to commit suicide was adjudicated on, and punished, for refusing to go into strip conditions (a practice that in itself is contrary to guidance issued by the Prison Service). These are practices which can flourish unchecked – not because of any wilful desire to abuse, but simply because they become customary.

In some prisons, we have found staff routinely reading all prisoners' personal correspondence – in one case because they thought it was helpful to know what was going on in their lives – in spite of ECHR rulings establishing prisoners' right to privacy and subsequent prison instructions that only a small proportion of correspondence should be randomly read, except for prisoners who pose specific risks.

Prison inspections are important for the small as well as the large things: for example, a Young Offender Institution which provided 18–20-year-old young men with a cold breakfast pack the night before – which unsurprisingly, was eaten before bedtime – and then only provided a baguette the following lunchtime, with no substantial meal until the evening; or a prison in which newly arrived prisoners were routinely 'squat-searched' over a mirror, in contravention of the governor's orders.

Inspections are also an opportunity to reveal and commend good practice: to point up prisons that are both humane and effective. Recently, we have inspected the three therapeutic communities, and two of the three resettlement prisons, in England. Those reports were overwhelmingly positive. They showed prisoners, many of them convicted of violent or serious offences, taking responsibility for themselves and their environment, without the usual structures – and in the case of resettlement prisons, without prison walls. We observed interchanges where prisoners and staff, on equal terms, were jointly trying to solve problems. These prisons offer an alternative to the coercive model, which simply responds to, and encourages, personal irresponsibility. But there are too few of them, and they need to take risks in a system which is inherently risk-averse.

The inspection of other forms of detention

We now regularly inspect Immigration Removal Centres, where immigrants and asylum-seekers who are not charged or convicted of criminal offences are held under administrative powers. Their detention is rightly subject to particularly high scrutiny. We found centres where detainees held in separation units, whether for disciplinary or protective reasons, were routinely strip-searched and held in strip conditions, without any assessment of risk. We have expressed particular concern about the detention of children, which we say should be exceptional and for no more than a matter of days. Yet when we inspected centres holding children, we found that there was no evidence of the minimum safeguards that should be in place to detain children and no independent assessment of the effect of detention on a child. Indeed, children appeared to be invisible to the authorities once the detention of their parents had been authorised. We found one autistic child who had not eaten properly for three days, and another who had been detained days before being due to sit his GCSE exams.

We do not routinely inspect court cells or prisoner escorts. When we did, in the course of area criminal justice inspections, we found, in one court, conditions that would not be tolerated within a prison: no certification of the number of prisoners who could be held in each cell, ineffective alarm bells and evacuation procedures, no child protection measures or risk assessments for carrying men, women and children in a single van. In another court recently, we found wooden partitioned cells 33 inches wide. They are now out of use.

Finally, we were recently asked to independently inspect the military corrective and training centre at Colchester, having already assisted the armed forces to develop procedures to manage detainees at risk of suicide. Given recent concerns about army facilities, both here and overseas, this is both welcome and necessary. We did not unearth any scandals, but we did find a failure to understand and implement the army's own policies on diversity. We also found a complaints procedure that did not meet international norms, or provide the necessary safeguards for detainees who might be at risk or vulnerable. All the detainees were marched on to the parade ground and called to attention by the company sergeant major. Anyone with a complaint was then invited to 'step out' and marched to a room where they could speak to the Army Visiting Officer, an officer from the nearby garrison.

The future of independent inspection

Those are examples of the way in which genuinely independent inspection lifts the lid on closed institutions on behalf of the public, pulls out common practices and exposes them to the light of what is normal and what is right. It is a very important protective and preventive measure. It is also an important driver for change, pointing out good practice, as well as bad, and giving ammunition to those running prisons, and supporting prisoners, to press for resources, support and reform.

But independent inspection of the kind that I have described can also be uncomfortable: for prisons, the prison service, officials and government. There is at present pressure to streamline and join up both public services and the structures that inspect them. There are undoubtedly gains to be made in making those services more efficient and accountable, reducing duplication, and filling in gaps in provision. Within criminal justice, there are evident gaps: among the different agencies charged with bringing offenders to justice and protecting communities; between those who look after people in prison and those who supervise them outside. But there is always a danger, in simplifying and amalgamating, that legitimately different aims and objectives are elided and confused.

We use the word 'inspection' to describe a variety of different functions: regulation, performance management, independent evaluation of whether public bodies are meeting standards and providing value for money. But the kind of inspection I have been describing is different. It is, as I said earlier, part of the system's 'ethical and community moorings'. It is no accident that we do not inspect the Prison *Service*, but the conditions in prisons and the treatment of prisoners. We examine the treatment of the prisoner as a whole person, not just an offender. We also examine the whole environment of the prison – healthcare, relationships, safety and education. And we need to do so in detail, establishment by establishment. There is a critical difference between inspection activity that examines the efficiency of the system as a whole, and that which provides a detailed and holistic account of each individual custodial environment. Finally, our work ranges beyond criminal justice to encompass other custodial settings, and reaches into those agencies and services that provide health, education, employment and housing for those in and after custody.

Independence is a fragile construct. It is, of course, important that it is set out in statute: that a Chief Inspector is responsible directly to the Secretary of State, not through any intermediaries or officials; that he or she has a duty to report as they find. But this is not enough. Before I was Chief Inspector, a delegation of Russians came to discuss prisons and prison policy. They asked about the inspectorate of prisons. 'Who appoints the Chief Inspector?' – 'The Home Secretary.' 'Where is the Chief Inspector's office?' – 'In the Home Office.' 'And who is the Chief Inspector?' – 'A retired General.' 'Ah,' they said in understanding tones. 'We too have independent inspectorates like that.'

It is the skirmishes around the edge of the territory, like the battle for our own standards, which often define the contours of independence. As in the nineteenth century, inspectors have constantly to be on the watch against becoming part of the system they inspect, however seductively that is presented by those who are part of it, and who may also genuinely wish to improve it.

Current proposals envisage prisons inspecting being subsumed into a 'justice and community safety' inspectorate, taking in the inspection of police, the prosecution service, the courts and probation, as well as prisons, and focusing on inspecting across the criminal justice system as a whole. Ministers have made clear that they wish the new body to retain a specific focus on inspection of places of custody, but the clear danger is that a human rights-based inspectorate will be peripheral to, and may become submerged within, a body whose main aims are the effectiveness of the criminal justice process and the reduction of crime. Those are laudable aims: but they are different, and require a different approach, methodology and focus.

I remain concerned that, over time and perhaps inadvertently, the sharp focus and robustly independent voice of the prisons inspectorate may be lost. One answer to the Russians' question is that, no matter what the background of the person you appoint, if you give them a remit to report independently and freely on the conditions in our overcrowded prisons, you leave them, and their inspection teams, no choice but to be robust, focused and at times awkward. But once that task is part of a broader aim, however necessary and laudable, there is a risk of blurring the process and changing the nature of the task and the way it is carried out.

I once said in a lecture:

> The bottom line is that, in reaching for new and innovative ways of solving old and so far intractable problems, we must not lose what we have got. That is a prisons inspectorate whose robust independence is a model for other countries; whose inspections and inspection methods are increasingly valued and adopted here; which is reporting on an alarmingly overcrowded and pressurised closed system; and which has responded to the challenge of expanding its custodial remit. This is an essential part of the protection of the human rights of those held in detention. It is too valuable to lose or diminish.

References

European Court of Human Rights (ECHR) (2002) www.echr.coe.int/Eng/Press/2002/mar/Edwardsjudepress.htm.

House of Lords (2003) Judgments – *Regina v Secretary of State for the Home Department* (Respondent) *ex parte* Amin (FC) (Appellant). www.publications.parliament.uk/pa/ld200203/ldjudgmt/jd031016/amin-1.htm.

House of Lords (2004) Judgments – *Regina v Her Majesty's Coroner for the County of West Yorkshire* (Appellant) *ex parte* Sacker (FC) (Respondent). www.parliament.the-stationery-office.co.uk/pa/ld200304/ldjudgmt/jd040311/sack-1.htm.

McConville S (1994) *English Local Prisons, 1860-1900. Next Only to Death*. Routledge, London.

Shaw J, Appleby L and Baker D (2003) *Safer Prisons: A National Study of Prison Suicides 1999-2000*. National Confidential Inquiry into Suicides and Homicides by People with Mental Illness. www.dh.gov.uk/assetRoot/04/03/43/01/04034301.pdf.

Chapter 16

Humane prisons: are they worth it?

Fiona Warren

We have a 'moral obligation' to treat our fellow beings, including offenders, humanely. In this chapter, democratic therapeutic community prisons are discussed as an example of humane imprisonment. This is legitimate insofar as the ideology underpinning the democratic TC (therapeutic community) approach can be seen to promote some basic aspects of humanity, such as the equal empowerment of individuals to register their view (usually in the democratic TC each member has one vote and all votes are of equal weight). A properly working democratic TC should be above debate about the humanity of its approach, as HMP Grendon has been seen to be (Genders and Player, 2004).

However, we could question whether it is *worth* using a democratic TC approach to do this. How do we *value* the humane or democratic TC prison? Hitherto, research into democratic TCs in prisons has comprised studies of the effectiveness of such interventions in which value is assessed in terms of reconviction rates and improvements in psychological functioning (Marshall, 1997; Shine, 2000; Shine and Hobson, 2000; Taylor, 2000). However, it would seem that the zeitgeist in offender programmes research is going to follow the trends within the NHS (National Health Service) in which there has been an emergent political imperative to establish the cost-effectiveness of interventions. A recent review exercise failed to find any studies of the cost-effectiveness of democratic TC prisons in UK (Warren *et al.*, 2005). It has been suggested that exploring the cost-effectiveness of democratic TCs (DTCs) in the prison system is now a high priority (Brand and Price, 2000).

There are many methodological, to put it politely, 'challenges' to conducting research into the effectiveness of any psychological/behavioural/social interventions. Research into the effectiveness of DTCs in prisons is beset with these and some additional ones of its own. Disappointment with the quality of research in high-security settings in general and high-security TCs in particular has been frequently voiced and the limitations of previous research methodology thoroughly discussed many times (Dolan and Coid, 1993; Warren *et al.*, 2003) although solutions have not been readily available.

Health economics is a whole field of specialist study which has gained sophistication and popularity relatively recently in science-year terms but remains a young discipline (Briggs, 2000). Reference to the health economics field shows that there are various approaches and complexities in evaluating the economics of delivering interventions. Within healthcare the solutions to date are not perfect and dissatisfaction remains with the quality of economic studies and their qualifications to be used to inform decision-making about resource use in the NHS (Barber and Thompson, 1998; Jefferson and Demicheli, 2002). Economic evaluations in the prison system are likely to borrow principles and methods from health economics, but applying these to prisons may well require adaptations and entail implications that are, as yet, unknown. Economic studies are likely to bring additional challenges to those already faced by clinical effectiveness studies of prison DTCs.

What economic analysis is designed to add to our knowledge that conventional studies of effectiveness (from here referred to as clinical effectiveness studies) do not, is consideration of the resources used to produce the outcomes we desire. Underlying the economic approach is the moral position that the world is comprised of a finite set of resources and that these ought to be deployed to maximum benefit. Using the health sector as an example, it can be seen that cost-effectiveness studies can be very important to therapeutic communities in meeting the political imperative. An example will serve to illustrate one way of conducting such a study and provide a platform for discussing the issues facing prison DTCs in exploring their cost-effectiveness.

One early approach to assessing the 'value' of DTCs in monetary terms was undertaken at Henderson Hospital. This is a residential DTC that offers treatment for up to one year for adults with personality disorder. It is the only non-prison DTC in the UK that does not combine treatment with psychotropic medication. Individuals enter treatment voluntarily and are able to leave treatment at any time. Although with a long history (it was founded in 1947) and respected in the TC world, the service was (and is) small, specialist and very different from mainstream psychiatry. At the time it was conducted, this particular study was extremely influential in determining local decisions about purchasing a threatened service, since it translated for relatively new health service commissioners the effects of this treatment, then perceived along with psychotherapy in general as 'an expensive luxury' (Holmes et al., 1994), into a cost-saving in their budget. This study was the first of its kind to be conducted on a UK DTC and is a very simple study – any future studies of this type in democratic TCs in prisons are likely to be expected to improve on this one considerably. The limitations of it are discussed below.

To set the context for the study: it arose following some policy changes to the structuring of funding of UK NHS services at the beginning of the 1990s. Services such as the Henderson Hospital were specialist (or tertiary) services in the NHS. The new funding arrangements required local contracts to purchase only a proportion of the service and for referrals from outside the jurisdiction of this contract to be negotiated on a patient-by-patient basis. The service set about considering the likely impact of this change and predicted difficulties for personality-disordered patients in gaining access to specialist treatment (Dolan and Norton, 1991). Indeed the predictions were fulfilled, with a 25 per cent reduction in referrals observed following the changes and with only just over one-third of funding requests made during the financial year receiving decisions within a month of the end of that financial year (Dolan and Norton, 1992). Research also demonstrated that 42 per cent of funding decisions were being made on other than clinical grounds (Dolan et al., 1994).

The study took place in two parts demonstrating two possible options for prison DTC research. In the first part, data were collected at baseline, and extrapolation from previous research was used to estimate (rather than directly measure) results. Data were collected on mental health and prison service usage on a sample of 29 (the number of places in the unit) consecutive admissions to the service. The data were collected from case notes and from forms routinely completed by admissions to the service. A sub-sample of 25 of the 29 also completed questionnaires about their service usage in the year prior to admission to the hospital. Costs were calculated by obtaining figures of extra-contractual referrals (ECR) tariffs for 1992–3 from the then four Thames Regional Health Authorities (RHA) (Table 16.1).

The daily tariff for Henderson Hospital at the time was £111 ($192) compared with £153.20 ($266) for a general acute psychiatric bed and £173 ($299) for Close Supervision Units. Prison was the cheapest resource at £386 ($669) per week. The 29 Henderson admissions had used a considerable amount of health and prison services in the previous year, the average estimated costs being £423 115 ($733 286) per year (mean cost per patient £14 590 ($25 285)). In this first part of the study, the cost of treatment at Henderson was offset by extrapolating from the lowest success rate (41 per cent) suggested by previous studies using service usage outcome measures (Copas *et al.*, 1984). The cohort of 29 patients were expected to stay in treatment for an average of seven months at a cost of £23 310 ($40 397) per patient or £675 990 ($1 171 535) for 29 patients. With a reduction of the annual bill post-treatment to 41 per cent (£173 477 or $300 647) this suggested that the treatment would 'pay for itself' in four years (Menzies *et al.*, 1993).

Subsequently, in the second part of the study (Dolan *et al.*, 1996), actual follow-up data had been obtained on actual service usage for 24 (83 per cent) of the 29 residents in the original sample (Table 16.2).

Information on service usage in the one year subsequent to discharge from Henderson was obtained from their referrer (in 17 cases) and/or their GP (in 14 cases) and from the client themselves (in 7 cases). Four participants had had further inpatient admissions, one of whom was re-admitted to Henderson. Two people had outpatient assessments, 12 had outpatient treatment and one attended a day hospital. None of the residents spent time in prison or a secure psychiatric unit during the year. The average cost of services used was £1308 ($2 266). The average actual cost of services used by these 24 residents in the one year prior to admission, using the data from the first study, had been £13 966 ($24 204). This represents an annual saving post-discharge of £12 658 ($21 937) per patient.

These 24 residents were in treatment at Henderson for an average of 231 days (range: 1 to 365 days). The actual cost of their treatment at Henderson was, therefore, £25 641 ($44 437). It was argued, successfully, that, should the cost of service usage continue at a similar rate for the years subsequent to the one year after discharge described by this study, the cost of admission to Henderson would be recouped in less than two years (rather than the four predicted) and represent savings to the public services budget in subsequent years.

Table 16.1 Service usage in the year before admission to Henderson: 24 patients at 1992–3 tariffs

Service	Units	No of patients	No of units	Unit mean £	Total cost £
Inpatient beds	Day	17	1568	153.2	240 218
Secure psychiatric beds	Day	2	140	173	24 220
Outpatient assessments	Each	6	6	179	1 074
Outpatient therapy	Episode	12	12	586	7 032
Day hospital	Day	3	404	71	28 684
Prison	Week	4	88	386	33 968
TOTAL COSTS					335 196
COST PER PATIENT					13 966

Table 16.2 Service usage in the one year following admission: 24 patients at 1993–4 tariffs

Service	Units	No of patients	No of units	Unit mean £	Total cost £
Inpatient beds	Day	3	73	179	13 962
Henderson Hospital	Day	1	50	110	5 500
Outpatient assessments	Each	2	2	166	,322
Outpatient therapy	Episode	12	12	790	9 480
Day hospital	Day	1	28	70	1 960
TOTAL COSTS					31 390
COST PER PATIENT					1 308

As acknowledged above, this study was very simple. The study demonstrates that cost studies of DTCs can be done in the NHS context and illustrates some of the issues for DTCs in prisons to consider in designing a cost study. This study also shows the importance of monitoring the effects of policy changes on DTCs, such as referral rates, as in this example. Changes in referral *types* or *sources* may be another effect that is observed.

As noted above, some of the methodological difficulties are common to both clinical and cost-effectiveness studies. Subsequent studies of other TCs in the health sector improved on this methodology in various ways but none of these represents a 'model' methodology for prison DTCs to adopt. There are some guidelines for evaluators of offender programmes produced by the Home Office summarising the steps involved in economic analysis and support is offered by the Home Office to complete the studies (Colledge *et al.*, 1999).

Box 16.1 Suggested steps in cost-effectiveness in the prison service

1 Define the intervention
2 Identify the inputs
3 Identify outputs and outcomes
4 Quantify inputs

5   Quantify attributable impacts and outcomes
6   Value inputs (costs)
7   Compare inputs with outputs and outcomes
Source: Colledge *et al.* (1999)

Sampling, sample size and response rate

The sample size in this study is very small. There is no reference to a calculation of statistical 'power' (the likelihood of the study being able to detect a difference if one is present) and, indeed, no statistics more compli-cated than a calculation of the mean were conducted on the cost data. It is common practice currently in the health sector to 'piggyback' cost-effective-ness analysis onto studies that are primarily of clinical effectiveness, as was the case in this example and as is recommended in a recent report regarding treatment for substance dependence in the prison system in England (Harrison *et al.*, 2003). This is seen as 'efficient' by researchers, who are 'killing two birds with one stone', and would be a tempting route for the prison DTC. However, one of the dangers is that, because of the nature of cost data (for example, they are often highly skewed and/or unclear) such studies are underpowered even if the clinical effectiveness study on the back of which they are sitting is appropriately powered (Briggs, 2000). (In contrast, if a combined study is appropriately powered for the cost analysis, it is likely to be 'overpowered' to test clinical effectiveness.) One danger of this is that studies which show a significant effect in their clinical outcomes and have a concomitant cost analysis that shows a reduction in cost or a lower cost than a comparison intervention without significance (or significance-testing) are interpreted as cost-effective interventions when, in fact, the question of cost-effectiveness has not actually been addressed, as in this case. For this reason, careful attention should be paid to the reporting of piggybacked cost-effectiveness studies, and confidence intervals rather than *p*-values should be used to express results, as is recommended in health; wide confidence intervals reveal when studies are underpowered (Altman and Bland, 1995). This issue of power is also an ethical one: should participants continue to be recruited for study after the intervention has been shown to be clinically effective (particu-larly if recruitment involves randomisation to the less effective comparison intervention) (Briggs, 2000)?

Achieving an acceptable sample size has implications for the research resources and feasibility of actually accomplishing the study. A recent paper on the feasibility of applying randomised controlled trial (RCT) methodology to the study of the efficacy of DTC prisons, in which offenders would be allocated at random to DTC prison or prison-as-usual, suggested that it would take nine years to complete such a study (Campbell, 2003). These calculations were done assuming reconviction as the outcome measure. Following the argument above, such a study would be likely to be insufficiently powered for a piggyback cost study and such a study would, therefore, take even longer than nine years to complete. Were several comparably operating DTCs to exist, adequate sample sizes could be recruited in less time (see below).

The use of informants other than the patients themselves in the Henderson study allowed for information to be gathered on a larger proportion of the sample than might have been obtained if data had only been collected from residents themselves. Information was thus obtained for 24 of the 29 people in the original study (83 per cent). However, only 7 of the clients (24 per cent) provided information, demonstrating neatly the consequences of relying on self-report data in studies. When only a small proportion of the invited sample responds, the degree to which results can be said to be true in general, rather than just true of people like the ones who responded to the study, is restricted. Depending on the types of data required (see below), the extent to which studies will need to rely on information given by offenders themselves will vary. However, it is recommended that information on other relevant aspects of an offender's life than reconviction is collected and there are many times when the offender themselves will be the only ones in possession of certain facts. There will always be a trade-off between the source of the data and its quality/quantity. Sometimes, as in this study, 'triangulation' of data collection (seeking the same information from more than one source) can be used, although this brings with it the problem of resolving contradictions between data sources.

It is good practice in quantitative research for data to be collected at comparable time points and in comparable contexts for each study participant, ideally prospectively. In the Henderson study the sample was of consecutive admissions but data were collected from these retrospectively. Studies of DTCs in the prison system can benefit from the fact that criminality data are routinely collected prospectively on all offenders by the police, Prison Service and Home Office and so lend themselves well to cost-effectiveness studies.

Comparison/control group and allocation

In this study there is no comparison or control group (participants were their own controls). We cannot infer that the changes shown were not due to something other than the treatment, such as the passage of time. Economic analysis is concerned with efficiency (a concept central to economic evaluation and more complex than this sentence implies!). Efficiency is a measure of whether resources are being used to get the best value for money (Williams, 1988). There are different types of efficiency (*see* Table 16.3) (Palmer and Torgerson, 1999) and the concept of 'perspective' is also central. The prison DTC cost evaluation is likely to need to address (*productive*) efficiency from the perspective of the criminal justice system. Productive efficiency entails giving priority to the provision of services that deliver the greatest benefit for the lowest cost (Palmer *et al.*, 1999). This contrasts with a societal perspective from which efficiency is achieved when resources are used such as to maximise the welfare of the society (so-called '*allocative efficiency*'). The DTC is therefore required to demonstrate that it is *more cost-effective than alternative approaches* to managing the kinds of offenders managed by prison

DTCs. Even to show *technical* efficiency (that they were producing certain levels of outcome with the minimum resources) DTCs in prisons would need to make some comparison. This would be with themselves in a slightly different configuration of staffing or capital, for example. Policymakers are unlikely to be as interested in this level of efficiency.

Table 16.3 Types of efficiency

	Definition	*Prison TC examples*
Technical efficiency	The best outcomes are achieved with the specific resources available.	Does the DTC produce the best outcomes it can given the staffing and other resources? If the DTC did not have Wing Therapists, or if the inmates stayed for less time, would the reoffending rate be higher?
Productive efficiency	The maximum health outcomes are achieved for a given cost *or* given outcomes are produced for the minimum cost.	The DTC is the cheapest intervention that can produce a reduction of reoffending of x.
Allocative efficiency	Resources are being allocated to maximise the welfare of society.	Society benefits maximally if x resources are spent on providing DTC treatment for offenders.

In the prison sector, comparison groups for study are also an important but difficult research challenge which has been discussed by those who have conducted reconviction studies of DTCs (Marshall, 1997; Shine, 2000; Taylor, 2000). Given that the therapy in the DTC is seen to be delivered via the whole configuration of the system and institution (rather than in a discrete set of therapeutic interventions occurring weekly, for example), the most appropriate comparison group is likely to be a sample of prisoners in the mainstream prison system. However, offenders differ widely and the issue of appropriate matching variables does not have a clear answer although aspects that have been considered include: age, sentence length, severity of index offence, offence history, socio-demographic/social aspects.

There remains a division in the research field with some arguing that a randomised controlled trial is inappropriate and/or meaningless in the context of a DTC and others arguing that it is unethical not to do one. However, feasibility studies (such as Campbell, 2003) suggest that the resources required to conduct RCTs are likely to be prohibitive whether or not the methodological debate is resolved.

Control over the interventions offered

It is widely acknowledged in the 'TC world' that institutions bearing the name TC can vary considerably (Kennard, 1998) and the culture of a healthy TC can be difficult to describe and to sustain (Norton, 1992). It cannot be assumed that just by virtue of calling itself a TC a regime is embodying the humane principles underlying a TC. Differences between institutions bearing the name TC include variations in ways that could be considered very important to their therapeutic potential. The TC from which the, remarkably often cited, view that psychopathic prisoners deteriorate as a result of TC intervention is a good example (Harris *et al.*, 1994; Warren, 1994).

In addition DTCs are 'complex interventions' (Manning, 2004) because they rely on group methods and the peer group as the primary agents of change. They are not manualised, although there are descriptions and processes that attempt to deliver quality control such as the Community of Communities project and the accreditation system (Haigh and Tucker, 2003; HM Prison Service, 2004b). The difficulty of controlling what is delivered limits the generalisability of results about one TC to others or to the same TC at a different time. This is a particular concern for randomised controlled trial methods (Wolff, 2001) and there is, as yet, no solution to this except to treat the time spent in the TC as a 'black box'. Similarly, in the comparison group of offenders in mainstream prison, there will be a methodological need to, but a pragmatic difficulty with, controlling (and possibly identifying) the experiences and interventions received.

Follow-up time

The extent of follow-up is also a key concern. Although some argue that follow-up should be as long as possible (Davies and Menzies, 2004) and studies of reconviction are constantly attempting to extend their follow-up periods, it is also the case that the more time that elapses between the intervention and the follow-up assessment, the greater the opportunity for other factors to influence that assessment. However, follow-up should at least include assessment after individuals have left the DTC and have had a 'fair period' at risk in the outside world.

Outcome measures: what is costed and how?

The outcome measure(s) selected should be related to the aims of the treatment (Norton and Dolan, 1995). There remains some debate about the primary aims of the DTC in the prison context, whether these are to reduce criminogenic risk or to increase psychological wellbeing (Blackburn, 2004) and the accreditation literature currently suggests both (HM Prison Service, 2004a). With complex cases such as people with personality disorders and the offenders who attend DTC prisons, there are many potential outcomes that could be relevant and no one comprehensive measure that assesses them all.

In this example, a selection of resources was chosen for measurement on the basis of relevance and pragmatism. In this case, data were collected regarding psychiatric inpatient and outpatient service use and prison stays. These are undoubtedly crude units of data. In their favour they could be argued to represent the most 'severe' service usage: we would hope that people were not re-admitted to acute psychiatric hospitals for long stays and certainly that they were not sentenced to prison following specialist treatment in the DTC. In fact, in this case, simply measuring those resources did show what seems to be a substantial reduction. Of course (as noted above), no tests of statistical significance were conducted on these figures. However, it is well known that personality-disordered patients use a wide range of services other than mental health and prison. Social work, accident and emergency, probation, GP and non-statutory services were not costed by this study but all are used more by personality-disordered patients than by the average member of the general population.

In the context of DTC prisons, previous studies have primarily focused on reconviction rates after leaving the TC. Whilst these have advantages in terms of response rate and hence representativeness, they can be argued to be a crude measure since the true picture of reoffending is mediated by the 'clear-up' rate of the police forces and the processes of the courts. In addition, there may be more 'subtle' changes in the offender and his/her behaviour that can only be measured by looking at social integration, employment, reductions in interpersonal aggression and improvements in family relationships, including parenting. The prison service recommends that existing and routinely collected sources of data are used for cost studies (Colledge et al., 1999).

There are three main approaches to economic evaluation (see Table 16.4) which differ in the way that they consider outcomes (or benefits) (Palmer, Byford et al., 1999). Cost-benefit analyses and cost-effectiveness studies allow other types of outcome to be measured. In the former kind of study, outcomes such as improvements in impulse control or social relationships are attributed a financial worth (this is controversial for obvious reasons and cost-benefit analyses have not flourished as a result) and in the latter type of study a ratio is produced of units of cost required to produce units of benefit. A third alternative is the cost-utility study in which the benefits measured include quantity and quality of health such as quality of life years (QALYS) which overcomes the problem posed by having many relevant outcomes in this population (Rehm et al., 2000). In addition, one solution to the conversion of health benefits to economic values that has been proposed is the idea of 'willingness to pay'. However, it is not clear how this would be determined in respect of DTC treatment for offenders. Who would decide what society was willing to pay for the outcomes achieved and how would they decide this – on the basis of clinical effectiveness studies, perhaps? Or by considering the cost of crime? In the example study, the analysis of reductions in costs did not employ any 'discounting principle' in which the opportunity cost, of spending the money and deriving the benefits sooner rather than later, is taken into account (Torgerson and Raftery, 1999). In addition, although it was persuasive, one of the additional problems with the example study (and with any future cost studies of DTCs in prisons) is that no real money is saved (Rehm et al., 2000) since the usage of resources is not actually changed by the activities of a small subsection of the population, such as those offenders who attend a DTC.

Table 16.4 Types of economic evaluation study

		Description
1	Cost-benefit	Benefits are expressed in monetary terms. Various interventions or scenarios can be compared.
2	Cost-effectiveness	Benefits are measured naturally. A ratio is produced of cost per unit of benefit (e.g. years of life saved, reduction in blood PSA levels).
3	Cost-utility	Benefits are measured in terms of quantity and quality of health (e.g. Quality of Life Years (QALYs)).

Summary

In summary, the areas of good research practice illustrated by the early economic study of Henderson that could be adopted by prison DTCs and areas that clearly need improvement are as follows. A suggested checklist for design issues for economic evaluations in DTCs in prisons is in Table 16.5. The areas of good practice demonstrated are: the collection of post-treatment data from independent sources (e.g. GPs and referring clinicians, central databases of criminal activity), which is likely to both increase follow-up rate and avoid biases in response (towards 'faking good or bad', inherent in patient/client report) or in the selection of the follow-up sample arising from clients who are either more positive about the unit (or more negative) being more motivated to respond to such a study; clear presentation of the units counted; the cost of each of these (unit cost). Studies presenting results only in one form, such as the total costs of resource use, prohibit comparison with other studies or other times (Bateman and Fonagy, 2003).

Table 16.5 Checklist of issues in design

• Sampling and representativeness of the sample of the population	Is the response rate sufficient? What is the sample representative of? Is the study powered appropriately to answer questions about cost-effectiveness?
• Control group for comparison	Matched sample from mainstream prison system. On which characteristics should matching occur? Should this include time of release? How will these offenders be identified?
• Allocation to treatment or control	Is randomisation scientifically ideal? Ethical? Feasible? What are the implications – time, resources?
• Measure of outcome	Reoffending (hard to measure accurately, not equal to reconviction)? Psychological benefits? Contributions to society via employment, etc.?
• Control of the interventions delivered	DTCs are complex interventions that rely on multiple processes with multiple individuals over a long period of time (difficult to control)

Table 16.5 (*cont.*)

• Thorough and relevant assessments of participants	Interdependent with the aims of treatment. Assessment of criminogenic need, personality and other psychological variables, previous resource use.
• Length of follow-up	Ideally post intervention, no agreement about how long. Home Office recommends two years

Studies of NHS DTCs that have attempted to improve on this methodology have done so by allocating patients to treatment versus comparison groups using non-clinical criteria (such as geography) (Chiesa *et al.*, 2002), although none have used a randomised design; recruiting larger sample sizes and achieving a higher response rate (Chiesa *et al.*, 2002); gaining data regarding service usage pre-treatment from routinely collected sources rather than self-reports from clients or clinicians (Davies and Campling, 2003). A more recent study of the cost of Henderson Hospital improved on previous methodology by attempting to cost a wider range of services and including in the costing of Henderson treatment additional services used during treatment (such as visits to the local Accident and Emergency department) (Fiander *et al.*, 2004). Whilst these subsequent studies represent improvements in many ways, they also suffer significant methodological flaws of their own, however, and none is a perfect role model for the DTC in prison.

Conclusions

We do not yet know the answer to the question whether humane prisons are *worth* it in financial terms at the moment and the way in which DTCs in prisons might respond to the imperatives to assess their cost-effectiveness is not straightforwardly clear. It would not seem advisable to simply adopt research models from democratic TCs in the NHS since the quality and sophistication of research designs have increased since these were conducted and DTCs within prisons have characteristics (of context and population) that differ importantly from those in the NHS. However, the NHS DTC studies do provide a platform from which to consider improvements, and replication of these methodologies may represent a pilot attempt in the prison context to address cost-effectiveness issues. In addition, some principles for good research practice in cost studies within the health sector are emerging and further discussion is needed to clarify how best DTCs can respond to these. One of the current difficulties with implementing economic studies of interventions is the lack of available expertise to accomplish this (Rehm *et al.*, 2000). We should perhaps not underestimate the need for this expertise and should requisition it where possible! It is unlikely that a cost study of DTCs that is conducted by researchers without expertise in economic analysis and which is blindly piggybacked on a clinical effectiveness study will be informative.

References

Altman DG and Bland JM (1995) Statistics notes: Absence of evidence is not evidence of absence. *BMJ*. **311**(7003): 485.

Barber JA and Thompson SG (1998) Analysis and interpretation of cost data in randomised controlled trials: review of published studies. *BMJ*. **317**(7167): 1195–200.

Bateman A and Fonagy P (2003) Health service utilization costs for borderline personality disorder patients treated with psychoanalytically oriented partial hospitalization versus general psychiatric care. *American Journal of Psychiatry*. **160**(1): 169–72.

Blackburn R (2004) 'What works' with mentally disordered offenders. *Psychology, Crime and Law*. **10**(2): 297–308.

Brand S and Price R (2000) *The Economic and Social Costs of Crime*. Home Office Research Study 217. Research, Development and Statistics Directorate, Home Office, London.

Briggs A (2000) Economic evaluation and clinical trials: size matters. *BMJ*. **321**(7273): 1362–3.

Campbell S (2003) *The Feasibility of Conducting an RCT at HMP Grendon*. Home Office Online Report, London. www.homeoffice.gov.uk/rds/pdfs2/rdsolr0303.pdf.

Chiesa M, Fonagy P, Holmes J *et al*. (2002) Health service use costs by personality disorder following specialist and non-specialist treatment: a comparative study. *Journal of Personality Disorders*. **16**(2): 160–73.

Colledge M, Collier P, Brand S *et al*. (1999) *Programmes for Offenders: guidelines for evaluators*. Research, Development and Statistics Directorate, Home Office, London.

Copas JB, O'Brien M, Roberts J *et al*. (1984) Treatment outcome in personality disorder: The effect of social, psychological and behavioural variables. *Personality and Individual Differences*. **5**: 565–73.

Davies S and Campling P (2003) Therapeutic community treatment of personality disorder: service use and mortality over 3 years' follow up. *British Journal of Psychiatry*. **182**(Supplement 44): s24–7.

Davies S and Menzies D (2004) Economic evaluations in therapeutic community research. In: J Lees, M Manning, D Menzies and N Morant (eds) *A Culture of Enquiry: research evidence and the therapeutic community*. Jessica Kingsley, London.

Dolan BM and Coid J (1993) *Psychopathic and Antisocial Personality Disorders: treatment and research issues*. Gaskell, London.

Dolan BM, Evans C, Norton K *et al*. (1994) Funding treatment of offender patients with severe personality disorder: Do financial considerations trump clinical need? *Journal of Forensic Psychiatry*. **5**: 263–74.

Dolan BM and Norton K (1991) The predicted impact of the NHS bill on the use and funding of a specialist service for personality disordered patients: A survey of clinicians' views. *Psychiatric Bulletin*. **15**: 402–4.

Dolan BM and Norton K (1992) One year after the NHS Bill: The extra-contractual referral system at Henderson Hospital. *Psychiatric Bulletin*. **16**: 745–7.

Dolan BM, Warren FM, Menzies D *et al*. (1996) Cost-offset following specialist treatment of severe personality disorders. *Psychiatric Bulletin*. **20**: 413–17.

Fiander M and Langham S (2004) *Henderson Replication Study, Clinical Progress and Health Economic Strands*. Final Report submitted to the National Programme on Forensic Mental Health R&D, London.

Genders E and Player E (2004) Grendon: A therapeutic community in prison. In: J Lees, M Manning, D Menzies and N Morant (eds) *A Culture of Enquiry: research evidence and the therapeutic community*. Jessica Kingsley, London.

Haigh R and Tucker S (2003) *Community of Communities: interim report and reflections on the process of this community.* www.therapeuticcommunities.org/community-of-communities.htm.

Harris G, Rice M, Cormier CA *et al.* (1994) Psychopaths: is the therapeutic community therapeutic? *Therapeutic Communities* **15**: 283–300.

Harrison L, Cappello R, Alaszewski A *et al.* (2003) *The Effectiveness of Treatment for Substance Dependence within the Prison System in England: a review.* Centre for Health Services Studies, University of Kent, Canterbury.

HM Prison Service (2004a) Democratic Therapeutic Communities: Core Model. (Unpublished.)

HM Prison Service (2004b) Democratic Therapeutic Communities: Core Model. Theory Manual. 1–80. (Unpublished.)

Holmes J and Marks I (1994) Psychotherapy – a luxury the NHS cannot afford? *BMJ.* **309**: 1070–1.

Jefferson T and Demicheli V (2002) Quality of economic evaluations in health care. *BMJ.* **324**(7333): 313–14.

Kennard D (1998) *An Introduction to Therapeutic Communities.* Jessica Kingsley, London.

Manning N (2004) The Gold Standard: what are RCTs and where did they come from? In: J Lees, M Manning, D Menzies and N Morant (eds) *A Culture of Enquiry: research evidence and the therapeutic community.* Jessica Kingsley, London.

Marshall P (1997) *A Reconviction Study of HMP Grendon Therapeutic Community.* Home Office, London.

Menzies D, Dolan BM, Norton K *et al.* (1993) Are short term savings worth long term costs? Funding psychotherapeutic inpatient treatment for personality disorders. *Psychiatric Bulletin.* **17**: 517–19.

Norton K (1992) A culture of enquiry: Its preservation or loss. *Therapeutic Communities: the International Journal for Therapeutic and Supportive Organizations.* **13**(1): 3–26.

Norton K and Dolan B (1995) Assessing change in personality disorder. *Current Opinion in Psychiatry.* **8**: 371–5.

Palmer S, Byford S, Raftery J *et al.* (1999) Economics notes: types of economic evaluation. *BMJ.* **318**(7194): 1349.

Palmer S and Torgerson DJ (1999) Economics notes: Definitions of efficiency. *BMJ.* **318**(7191): 1136.

Rehm J, Guggenbühl L, Uchtenhagen A *et al.* (2000) *Adequacy in Drug Abuse Treatment and Care in Europe. Part IV: Evaluations of effectiveness and economic evaluations.* WHO European Office and the Addiction Research Institute, Zurich.

Shine J (ed) (2000) *A Compilation of Grendon Research.* HMP Grendon.

Shine J and Hobson J (2000) Institutional behaviour and time in treatment among psychopaths admitted to a prison-based therapeutic community. *Medicine, Science and the Law.* **40**(4): 327–335.

Taylor R (2000) *A Seven-year Reconviction Study of HMP Grendon Therapeutic Community.* Research Findings No. 115. Home Office, London. Available at: www.homeoffice.gov.uk/rds/pdfs/r115.pdf.

Torgerson DJ and Raftery J (1999) Economics notes: Discounting. *BMJ.* **319**(7214): 914–15.

Warren F (1994) What do we mean by a 'Therapeutic community' for Offenders. *Therapeutic Communities* **15**(4): 312–18.

Warren F and Norton K (2005) *Research Analysis to Identify Future Research Needs in Prison Service Democratic Therapeutic Communities.* Report submitted to the Home Office.

Warren F, Preedy-Fayers K, McGanley G *et al.* (2003) Review of Treatments for Severe Personality Disorder. London, Home Office Online Publication. www.homeoffice.gov.uk/rds/onlinepubs1.html.

Williams A (1988) Priority setting in public and private health care. A guide through the ideological jungle. *Journal of Health Economics.* 7(2): 173-83.

Wolff N (2001) Randomised trials of socially complex interventions: promise or peril? *Journal of Health Services Research and Policy.* 6(2): 123-6.

Index